OVERCOMING THE COVID DARKNESS

OVERCOMING THE COVID DARKNESS

How Two Doctors Successfully Treated 7000 Patients

BRIAN TYSON, M.D. AND GEORGE FAREED, M.D.

With Mathew Crawford

Overcoming the COVID Darkness
How Two Doctors Successfully Treated 7000 Patients
Brian Tyson, M.D. and George Fareed, M.D.
With Mathew Crawford (Chapter 8)

Published by Brian Tyson, M.D. and George C. Fareed, M.D.
ISBN: 979-8-9855583-0-2

Disclaimer: The information presented in this book is the result of years of practice, experience, and clinical research by the authors. However, it is not a substitute for evaluation and treatment by a medical doctor. The information contained herein is for educational purposes only. It is not intended to be a substitute for professional medical advice.

The reader should always consult with his or her physician to determine the appropriateness of the information for his or her own medical situation and treatment plan. Reading this book does not constitute a physician-patient relationship. The stories in this book are true. The names and circumstances of the stories have been changed at times to preserve privacy.

DEDICATION

This book is dedicated to our wives, Fabiola and Martha, who have supported us throughout the pandemic, and to our children and grandchildren. We also dedicate it to all the many healthcare professionals and dedicated staff who stood by our sides to help all the patients achieve rapid and complete recoveries from effective, early COVID-19 therapy during 2020 and 2021.

Brian Tyson, M.D.   George Fareed, M.D.
El Centro, California   Brawley, California

THE AUTHORS' HOPE

It is our sincere hope this book helps more people understand the critical importance of early COVID-19 treatment because there may be harsh surges. If we have successfully treated and saved over 7,000 lives so far in our clinics and more than 1,200 in the Trinity Baptist Church C19 advocacy, then we hope this book might save many thousands more after that. We also hope that vaccination programs recognize that COVID-19 variants will continue to arise in those who have been vaccinated as long vaccines fail to completely block the infection.

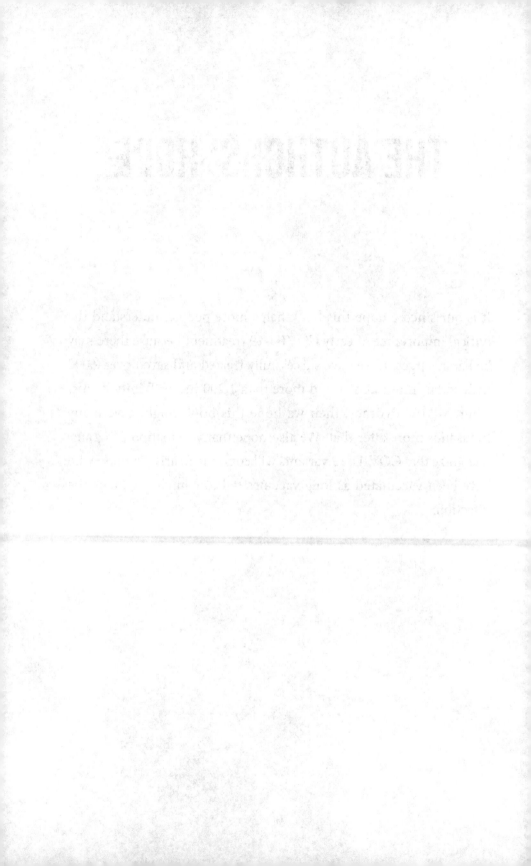

ACKNOWLEDGMENTS

The authors express their appreciation to Justice Hope, M.D., Donald Pompan, M.D., Michael Jacobs, M.D., Harvey Risch, M.D., Peter McCullough, M.D., Vladimir Zelenko, M.D., Sabine Hazin, M.D., Simone Gold, M.D., Joseph Ladapo, M.D., Ph.D., Robert Malone, M.D, Bruce Patterson, M.D., Robin Armstong, M.D., Jay Bhattacharya, M.D., Ph.D., Stella Immanuel, M.D., Ira Bernstein, M.D., Steven Hatfill, M.D., Pastor Richard Moore, Steve Kirsch, Jean-Pierre Kiekens, Sean Hannity, and Senator Ron Johnson for their support, inspiration, and advice to us throughout the pandemic.

The authors thank all of the doctors and medical staff at the All Valley Urgent Care clinics, the Public Health Department of Imperial County, CA, as well as the maintainers of the Imperial County COVID-19 data and associated tracking systems, for their help with this quality improvement study. We thank David Wiseman, Ph.D., for his review of the data and advice on various aspects of the study, as well as all of the doctors and researchers who have thoughtfully generated so much useful research during the pandemic. Our gratitude especially goes out to those whose insights into early ambulatory treatment protocols encouraged the practice of valuable care at All Valley Urgent Care and this analysis of the data.

We are indebted to Becky Hanks for early copy editing, Betty and Lloyd Miller (from *The Desert Review*), and Howard VanEs and his exceptional staff at Let's Write Books, Inc. for providing professional book writing, editing, and publishing services.

FOREWORD

BY JUSTUS R. HOPE, M.D.,

A physical medicine specialist and author from Modesto, CA

Some doctors are talented in their field and area of specialty. Others offer a compassionate bedside manner that puts their patients at ease instantly. It is uncommon, however, to find all of these qualities within the same person. Dr. George Fareed is one of those rare individuals who has both an inherent aptitude for medicine, along with patience, energy, and empathy for those in his care. While others might brag about their accomplishments, Dr. George Fareed remains a humble, soft-spoken man—despite an extensive list of accolades over the course of his distinguished career. This beloved small-town doctor, from the somewhat sleepy Imperial County in California, possesses a wealth of experience and an impressive education that have earned him the honor of being named the California Medical Association's Rural Physician of the year in 2015.

Words alone cannot express my respect and deep admiration for this man. The Dr. Fareed known by the world is the son of Dr. Omar John Fareed, a legend in his own time and a medical missionary who worked with Dr. Albert Schweitzer. He was a doctor with a heart who imbued those same values in his son, George.

The younger Dr. Fareed began his medical career with training at Harvard Medical School. After graduation, Dr. Fareed studied recombinant DNA and taught at Harvard and UCLA Medical Schools. He published research and eventually left academics for a job in the industry. While serving at XOMA Corporation and Advanced Antigens in biotech research, he developed processes that led to three U.S. patents.

Later, Dr. Fareed spent time following in his father's footsteps as a medical missionary in Africa. He clearly possesses that rare combination of altruism, empathy, and medical knowledge that is so sorely lacking in many of today's physicians. Like his father, Dr. Fareed also spent time as the Team Physician for the U.S. Davis Cup tennis teams, treating the greats like Andre Agassi, Pete Sampras, and Jim Courier.

In 1991, Dr. Fareed left academics for his true love: patients. He became a country doctor in the sleepy desert town of Brawley, California, where he became a pillar of its community. He served as the physician for the local football teams, while simultaneously treating the tennis stars. No matter the sport, he shared his legendary compassion with both. In fact, one of his high school student-athletes described Dr. Fareed as the "most compassionate doctor I have ever known."

Dr. Fareed also established the first HIV clinic in Brawley, and with incredible foresight, began administering cocktail drug treatments before it became the standard of care. Using repurposed drug cocktails to treat AIDS patients during that epidemic, Dr. Fareed certainly knows a thing or two when it comes to treating viruses, and he disagrees with those who say that even when used carefully, hydroxychloroquine (HCQ) is too dangerous to employ.

Not surprisingly, then, when the COVID-19 pandemic struck, and the Imperial Valley became the California epicenter, Dr. Fareed led the way out. Early in the pandemic, Dr. Fareed associated with Dr. Brian Tyson, a young urgent care center director from El Centro. Together, the two physicians led the nation in using repurposed drug cocktails to save virtually all of their patients. He and his colleagues have treated thousands of people with no ill effects, despite the media and the official positions against Hydroxychloroquine. But then again, Dr. Fareed is not your ordinary country doctor.

I was fortunate enough to cross paths with the impressive Dr. Fareed during my lifetime, and he has served as a mentor and colleague during a time when medicine has lost its ethics and forgotten the Hippocratic Oath. Dr. Fareed and Dr. Tyson—as well as Drs. McCullough, Risch, and Zelenko—are doctors who lead by example. An American hero, Dr. Zelenko is the person who formulated the treatment with HCQ, zinc, and azithromycin that saved hundreds of lives in New York State in March and April 2020. Dr. Peter McCullough is a cardiologist and internist from Dallas, TX, who published and presented widely on multidrug, sequenced early therapy since 2020. And last but not least, Dr. Risch is a professor of epidemiology at Yale University—not to mention being a champion for early treatment, based on his critical analyses. Dr. Risch actually called for this early treatment to be rolled out widely in May 2020 as well. Even today, these compatriots of medicine continue to shine the light of truth and science on one of our nation's darkest episodes.

I am honored to have been able to report on the doctors' fight to save patients' lives. I am also honored to have been included by

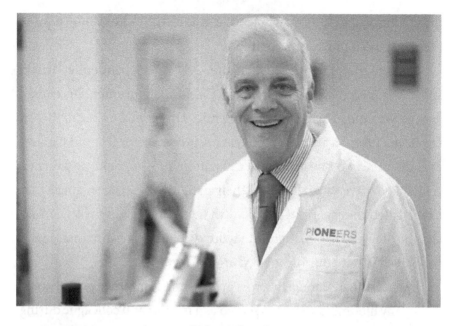

Dr. George Fareed

Dr. Donald Pompan, an orthopedic specialist, and Dr. Michael Jacobs, a family practice physician as fellow writers. This book details Dr. Fareed, Dr. Tyson, and his courageous colleagues' epic story—and I believe this true story will be recounted for generations. Just as Dr. Omar Fareed led young George by example, the example set by Dr. George Fareed during this pandemic will also inspire generations of future physicians.

* * *

Allow me now to describe Dr. Fareed's youthful associate. Dr. Brian Tyson, the fearless dynamo from El Centro, California, teamed up with Dr. Fareed to create the Miracle of the Imperial Valley: an epic story.

Dr. Tyson is a friend and colleague of Dr. Fareed who owns and operates All Valley Urgent Care in El Centro, California. El Centro is a border town located about twenty miles south of Brawley. Dr. Tyson has also already saved thousands of lives—and his commitment knows no bounds. In fact, at one point, Dr. Tyson took out a $250,000 personal loan to order personal protective equipment and COVID-19 testing supplies when he could not acquire them from the local health department or CDC.

Dr. Tyson is a no-nonsense doctor who practices in the trenches of COVID-19. He treats migrant farmworkers and meat-packing house employees who do not have the luxury of social distancing. In short, Dr. Tyson is a true warrior.

The team of Dr. Fareed and Dr. Tyson have now treated over 7,000 patients with COVID-19—and saved every one of them. Not a single death occurred while using early treatment. Only four hospitalizations happened under their watch, and unfortunately, they lost three individuals who presented to the clinic too late in the disease to be treated as an outpatient.

Did Dr. Tyson make medical history or win a Nobel Peace Prize? Did he receive the Presidential Medal of Freedom Award? No. Instead, he was informed his license might be in jeopardy if he continued treating patients with HCQ. Although this drug has been used safely for decades, it acquired a bad name through fraudulent citations of retracted studies, which you will learn more about within these pages. You can learn more about Dr. Tyson and his work with COVID-19 here: https://youtu.be/fe1TqxvXKTs.

Doctors rarely use terms like "miracle." It is considered unscientific by some, and I suppose other doctors might be worried about the criticism of using such a powerful word. However, during the

COVID-19 pandemic—when the FDA and CDC claimed there were no effective preventive measures or treatments for COVID-19, although two physicians documented almost 7,000 cases in a row of a real cure—the word "miracle" certainly comes to mind.

Drs. Tyson and Fareed's story is the stuff of legends. They saved thousands of lives through the use of repurposed drugs (old drugs already FDA-approved as safe for other diseases but useful in new ones, especially viruses like COVID-19 and even some terminal cancers). And whether it is politically correct or not, the time has come for repurposed drug cocktails to be used to save lives.

All Americans are guaranteed the right to "life, liberty, and the pursuit of happiness," regardless of the profit motive of corrupt governmental agencies. Drs. Tyson and Fareed deserve a Nobel Prize for.their work. This book contains their incredible true story.

October 2021
Justus R. Hope, M.D.
Physical Medicine & Rehabilitation
Redding, California

TABLE OF CONTENTS

INTRODUCTION

In late December 2019, the WHO (World Health Organization) country office located in China was notified of a cluster of viral pneumonia cases in Wuhan, China. However, little else was revealed, and there was minimal concern around the world. After all, viruses causing pneumonia, bronchitis, and other upper respiratory conditions are common in the medical field.

We expect these viruses to be ordinary. In most cases, we treat the patient with what is considered a classic protocol. Then, within a week to ten days, the patients improve, and life goes on a usual. But this virus was anything but ordinary—like nothing we have ever seen or experienced. We just didn't realize it at the time.

On January 24, 2020, patient samples obtained in Wuhan allowed the SARS CoV-2 virus to be identified and characterized for the first time. Days later, the WHO declared the SARS CoV-2 outbreak a Public Health Emergency of international concern. In the pandemic's infancy, from January through March 2020, new information sprouted up almost daily, as the world watched . . . and waited.

Keep in mind that, in those early days, there was no known effective treatment. In fact, many people were simply being told to go home from the hospital and "wait it out"—and only to return to the hospital if the virus became life-threatening. As we all know, in too many of these cases, returning to the hospital was too late for that person to recover and survive the deadly virus.

This approach had horrific consequences. Wait. Wait some more. Then, if you're *really* sick, go to the hospital, where you can be put on a ventilator. Then wait again and hope for a miracle. For far too many individuals, their miracle never showed up. Tragically, husbands, wives, mothers, fathers, and friends waited anxiously at home for word on their loved one's status in the hospital—without the ability to visit them or see them one last time.

If only they could have been tested early.

If only they could have received an effective treatment immediately —even before the test results were in.

If only.

This book exists because we found that a combination of hydroxychloroquine, zinc, and antibiotics could serve as an extremely effective treatment, if they were administered as early as possible. In fact, our results are nothing short of a *miracle*.

Despite the amazing success we achieved with more than 7,000 patients, all of the major medical organizations—from the WHO, to the NIH, to the CDC—did not welcome our information. Rather, they attempted to stop us from effectively treating patients, as well as suppress the information we knew the public needed to hear. We were even threatened with professional consequences if we were to continue providing this life-saving treatment to COVID-positive individuals.

Why? Why would anyone want to *stop* getting the word out, when a pandemic that rocked the globe could be effectively treated? Why would doctors on the front lines, saving lives each day, be threatened with punishment from their own colleagues?

Consider this: when the world was desperate to find a treatment or cure for a deadly disease, and when we actually provided that information . . . it was censored. Most people would say, WTF? But we wouldn't give up. In fact, we channeled our anger into collective action, by publishing a raw video of speeches that spoke the truth . . . and then posting and reposting again, as the videos were repeatedly taken down.

Despite the pushback, we won't stop posting, until it is recognized all over the world that we do not need to be afraid anymore. People need to know—and be reassured—that we *will* survive this pandemic, just like pandemics of the past. There *is* treatment available. This treatment works when used early, and it is highly effective.

In this book, you will learn more about our roles as doctors, as the COVID-19 pandemic spread across the world and we effectively tested and treated thousands of patients. We will describe what we did to help our patients, how we saved lives, and the information we shared with other medical professionals.

We will share our journey, from a perhaps naïve optimism that this treatment would be met with open arms, to the struggle we faced in getting the word out to the public, amidst suppression and censure from politicians and even others in the medical profession.

Despite making congressional statements, providing data to prove our success rates, and thousands of anecdotal stories of treatment and recovery, the CDC, NIH, or any other medical organization would not listen. They were too busy telling the public that there was no cure.

In this book, you'll read testimonials, articles from newspapers and other media, excerpts from medical studies, interview transcripts, transcripts from congressional hearings, and presentations made to various organizations. You will also discover what other doctors around the world are saying about this highly successful treatment.

Plus, you will hear real patients' stories that will help you better understand why the work we have done demands to be heard.

Our voices *will* be heard . . . because we hear the cry of those in our care. Physicians are people too; we have families and kids. We would never advocate for something in which we did not believe.

I believe many scientists are different; financial gains and incentives may complicate their decision-making process. In addition, there are research funding needs and pressures, and while they may have the best of intentions, these scientists do not work on the frontlines. They do not care for patients; they do not need to explain the risks and benefits of treatments to families. They are not there when patients break down and cry because they have tested positive. They don't have to explain to a nine-year-old girl that she will not kill her parents just because she tested positive. Scientists, on the other hand, have no vested interest or experience with real people and families—and no emotional pain when things do not go their way.

This virus has killed people! It will kill more. The question is, how many more will die unnecessarily from not receiving the available treatment? How many will die in fear, and how many will die alone?

Our final point is this: when you get sick, you do not go to the CDC or the NIH. You don't call the U.S. Food and Drug Administration to receive a diagnosis and treatment. Where do you go? You go to your doctor! You go to the people who have seen a disease before and know how to treat it. This virus is no different.

We invite you to witness our journey, and how we accomplished a miracle. The world needs to know the real story of COVID-19: the good, the bad, and the ugly. Everyone deserves to know the truth— and the truth is far different from what you have heard from Dr. Fauci or in the media. In the pages that follow, we share our experience.

CHAPTER 1

MEET DR. FAREED
AND DR. TYSON

This is the story of two medical doctors trying to do the best work possible to alleviate suffering in the face of a terrifying viral illness inflicted on the world. While we had worked together in a professional capacity before, nothing quite prepared us for the journey we would embark on together when China released the COVID-19 virus at the end of 2019.

As medical professionals, we came together to develop a successful scientific and medical approach to the pandemic. And even though we had major obstacles to overcome, we persevered to find solutions, despite the ongoing lack of proper guidance from official national and international sources for what should be (and should have been) done to combat the pandemic.

FROM DR. FAREED: MOVING TO THE IMPERIAL VALLEY AND MEETING DR. TYSON

I graduated with honors from Harvard Medical School in 1970 and pursued academic and research work at the NIAID and as faculty both at Harvard and UCLA. In 1991 I left the academic and biotechnology worlds that consumed me for nearly 20 years to pursue my true calling in medicine for family medicine in an underserved region of California called the Imperial Valley. During that time in 1992, I created HIV services for the Valley, as I had realized there was a dire need for early treatment with antivirals to alleviate the advancement of HIV to AIDS. Little did I know at the time, but my experience with antivirals would become critical thirty years after I created those services—but this time for treating COVID-19. It was also during my time in the Imperial Valley that I met Dr. Brian Tyson.

FROM DR. TYSON: TEAMING UP WITH DR. FAREED

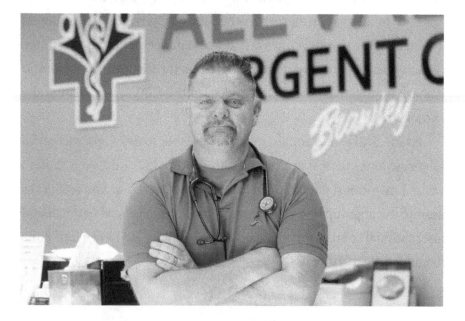

Dr. Brian Tyson

6

Dr. Fareed and I worked together for many years in Brawley, California, at the local hospital, Pioneers Memorial Healthcare District Hospital. In addition to my work at the hospital, I had established a clinic in El Centro, California: the All Valley Urgent Care Clinic. Periodically, Dr. Fareed would give me a much-needed break by working shifts at my clinic during the years preceding the pandemic of 2020. With the onset of COVID-19, Dr. Fareed continued working both in outpatient care and as a hospitalist (in-patient physicians who work exclusively in a hospital) periodically, treating inpatient cases that had progressed to respiratory failure and required mechanical ventilation. Dr. Tyson was exclusively working in his urgent care center.

When the pandemic became a reality in March 2020, both of us elected to use an agent that had previously been shown to be an effective antiviral against coronaviruses like COVID-19. Hydroxychloroquine (HCQ) had already been in use in France when Dr. Didier Raoult—Director of the Infectious Disease Center in Marseille, France, and a world-renowned specialist in tropical diseases and infectious diseases—produced what appeared to be excellent benefits for preventing hospitalization and death. The protocol for its use in New York by Dr. Vladimir "Zev" Zelenko, a family practice physician in upper New York who pioneered the early use of hydroxychloroquine, zinc, and azithromycin, showed encouraging results as well. We decided to use HCQ in a protocol utilizing a somewhat higher dose, but nothing at all toxic or dangerous.

Most of the protocols used the HCQ in doses of approximately 2400 milligrams over five to eight days. In our protocol, we utilized HCQ at 3200 mg over five days of treatment (based on the higher dosages Dr. Raoult was using). We found the key for effective treatment was employing the protocol with this antiviral agent in the early phase of the infection of COVID-19—no later than ten to fourteen days of infection, and preferably within the first three to five days.

In the early months of the pandemic, we saw in both the urgent care and Brawley clinics at the Pioneers Hospital hundreds and hundreds of symptomatic adult patients in need of early treatment to prevent the consequences of viral spread and damage in the lungs and other major organs.

Due to totally inappropriate and severely lacking guidelines from the CDC, FDA, and Dr. Fauci, emergency rooms were quickly inundated with symptomatic patients. Without a proper protocol, patients were being sent home to fight off the viral infection with no appropriate antiviral therapy—only to return when they experienced severe respiratory distress, requiring hospitalization with probable intubation and placement on mechanical ventilation.

We felt this "protocol" was a cruel and heartless action that unfortunately impacted most medical practitioners in outpatient centers, ERs, and hospitals. International medicine relied upon guidance from the United States, resulting in a tidal wave of acceptance for doing nothing. It was nihilism. The growing numbers of fatalities and long-term injuries in those who should have recovered from their hospital ordeals were exceptionally depressing to us.

But it wasn't just in the hospital setting where people were dying en masse. With outbreaks in assisted living centers, we knew our treatment was critical to saving the lives of the elderly—some of the most vulnerable among us.

Unfortunately, instead of receiving encouragement for our work, we faced criticism. In fact, we were even threatened with professional sanctions if we continued our life-saving protocols. Despite those threats, we persisted, as we saw too many other professionals in our field stand idly by, watching patients needlessly die in their care.

Fortunately, being in a rural area detached us somewhat from academic influences. This gave us the freedom to do what we knew worked (as opposed to taking the wait-and-see advice at face value as the only option). By following our effective protocol, were also able to witness extraordinary improvements and the resolution of symptoms in our patients. The gratitude and testimonials we have received have been prolific, and we know in our hearts that there is no reason for doctors to modify successful and life-saving treatments just to pacify the naysayers, pessimists, and unbelievers brainwashed by national agencies.

Sadly, some medical academics published patently false information early on, which you will learn more about in this book. Many flawed clinical trials were guided and published by individuals with vast conflicts of interest. Unfortunately, their ulterior motives were never disclosed. To appease these fraudulent academics, medical institutions and official agencies essentially blocked all early treatment protocols using HCQ.

Even though that false information was later retracted, the damage was done: our work was being discounted, and people continued to believe misinformation as they blindly accepted certain doctors' recommendations as gospel.

Meanwhile, we couldn't bear to witness the dire consequences of withholding treatment—not as we saw other patients go into respiratory failure and die on ventilators alone, without the basic human right of having their loved ones by their side.

We knew at our core that what we were doing was right—because it *worked*. In fact, the gratitude and outpouring of support we have received has been both humbling and yet another affirmation of our commitment to continue to get the word out.

Is the mainstream media the end-all and be-all for truth? Or are ulterior motives and politics putting our lives in jeopardy, as if we are pawns in a life-or-death game of chess? Consider just a few of our patients' stories, as they were told to reporters of *The Desert Review* and *Calexico Chronicle*, and decide for yourself:

- Jim Hanks, age seventy-four, is a well-known local figure in the Imperial Valley. When Hanks began experiencing symptoms of respiratory complications from COVID-19, his cousin reached out seeking help from Dr. Fareed.

  "People in the U.S. don't have to die because others hate the President," Hanks said. This, after Hanks had been discharged from the emergency room to basically fight it off at home or come back when he could not breathe.

  "I can't say enough about Dr. Fareed. I am living proof his protocol works, and I took it late. In prescribing the medications, Dr. Fareed explained precisely how they would affect me and when I should start feeling better. He was spot on, including oxygen levels and body temperature."

  As for cost? That week's dose of the prescribed medicine cost him a mere $37.

- Another couple, Charlie and Meg Slater, said, "We reached out to Dr. George Fareed for advice, [and] he directed us to go immediately to the PMH drive-through COVID testing site at his clinic. This was at 8 AM. By 9:30 AM, Dr. Fareed was calling my wife with the results: we both tested positive for COVID. He immediately made arrangements for us to go to the Emergency Room at PMH for the monoclonal infusions, as well as instructing us to begin taking his 'COVID Cocktail' protocol."

Charlie explained that initially there were "no head cold symptoms for my wife, although I still had a bit of a chest cough. The next few days followed with extreme fatigue, and finally [we lost] our sense of taste and smell, so we rested." Two days after the infusions, both noticed a significant improvement and felt "back to normal," despite Charlie's history of serious health problems over the last few years.

- Imperial resident Dionte Bell said he thinks he caught COVID while either working the vehicle lanes or the pedestrian lanes at the Calexico West Port of Entry in early July 2020.

After getting to the point where he already had no taste, experienced shortness of breath, a blinding headache, and a fever that would not go away, he walked into the ER at Pioneers Memorial Hospital on Sunday, July 12, 2020.

A healthy man, who regularly lifts weights and exercises, Bell took a COVID test and was told to go home and isolate until the results came back. He wasn't given any medication and didn't get any results back until July 14th or 15th.

As he began feeling worse, he called his physician on July 22nd—ten days after being tested, and Dr. Fareed immediately called in a five-day course of the HCQ cocktail.

"It felt really strong at the beginning; it made my heartbeat rise," Bell remembers. "But after a day or two, I got used to it."

What amazed Bell, though, was the very night he began taking the cocktail, he could feel his symptoms start to subside, his fever relented, and his headache went away.

These are real people we treated, along with thousands more. Check out their stories (links to the stories at the end of this book), and ask yourself whom you plan to listen to: those in the ivory tower with theories that ask you to do nothing but "wait and see" how much COVID affects your body . . . or listen to those on the frontlines who are providing early, effective treatment—and saving 100% of their patients' lives, when caught within the early stages?

This book is based on our long, arduous journey. Our battle is for truth, while shielding our patients and the world from dishonesty, incompetence, conflicts of interest, and inhumanity.

CHAPTER 2
THE PANDEMIC BEGINS
(January – April 2020)

We heard about the Wuhan Virus in January of 2020. And like everyone else at the time, we thought it was simply another outbreak in China, like the bird flu or influenza. At first, it did not appear to be anything worrisome. But when we realized that Chinese healthcare providers were getting sick—followed by the Wuhan physician who died—we suddenly took notice. We knew that, due to international travel, it was only a matter of time before the virus would make its way to the U.S.

FROM DR. FAREED: FROM CALM TO FEAR

My wife and I went on vacation in February 2020, before travel restrictions were instituted in the United States and other countries from the COVID-19 pandemic. At that time, all appeared to be calm and safe, and we were all following the declarations from Dr. Fauci, indicating there was not much to worry about regarding the impact of the COVID -19 in the United States.

During our vacation, Martha and I enjoyed scuba diving in the Sea of Cortez and sailing among the beautiful islands near the town of Loreto, Mexico. However, upon our return to Imperial Valley in the latter part of February, it became quite clear that COVID-19 was already infecting people in our local area, and cases were coming in from Mexico across the border from the rural southeastern area of California.

FROM DR. TYSON: FROM FEAR TO ACTION

I told my wife, "We need to get prepared, and we are going to need a plan."

During this time, I remember getting a call from my daughter Mahkenna's music manager, Gary Salzman, whom she was supposed to fly out and visit in late March about her new single.

Gary told me, "I think I have this crap!"

I replied, "How do you feel? Is it bad?"

He said, "It's in my lungs, and I'm having a hard time breathing."

I suggested he go to the ER and get tested to be sure and then, if he were positive, to receive available treatment. I had already been doing some research from studies by Dr. Didier Raoult coming out of southern France. A study published by the Journal of Virology in 2005 showed chloroquine was a potent inhibitor of SARS coronavirus infection and spread, so I told him to get on hydroxychloroquine, zinc, and a Z-pack.

His response was that, after visiting the ER, they sent him home with no treatment. They said he was not even sick enough to get a test for the virus. Without the ability to test, his treatment as an outpatient was withheld. It wasn't until he became sicker and later ended up in the hospital that they paid any attention to him.

Gary died two weeks later.

We were devastated as a family, the music community lost a legend, and we could not even have a proper funeral for him. In that moment, I told myself I would not allow this tragedy to happen with any of my patients. I would find a way to test people and treat people when that day came.

The media and President Trump initiated press conferences to notify the U.S. citizens that the virus was a real concern, and they wanted to shut down travel from China to the United States. Due to the political nature of what was going on, I witnessed something I had never seen before: I saw the Democratic party, at the time, insisting that anything Donald Trump did was wrong. Yet they offered no solutions to the contrary. This was the beginning of the political game that led to countless unnecessary deaths in our country.

While the president was forming his team and trying to implement a protection plan, Nancy Pelosi was out in Chinatown, proclaiming how safe it was and inviting everyone to visit and enjoy the festivities. Dr. Fauci, Trump's advisor, was claiming the outbreak was no more dangerous than a normal flu, and he did not believe the U.S. needed a travel ban or to make any real preparations.

The mainstream media was also weighing in, calling the president xenophobic for wanting to ban travel. It was ugly political mudslinging in the beginning stages of what would become the largest pandemic since the Spanish Flu.

It was difficult to understand why the virus had to become a political issue. When have medicine and healthcare been political? We can only relate this to the pro-life and pro-choice issues as the only other existing political-medical fights.

Both parties have distinct versions of what healthcare coverage should look like, regarding prescription drug plans and right-to-try issues. However, we have never had such a polarizing discussion on how best to protect our country with suggested policies that are not based on true science.

How does one politically disagree with science? A virus is not political. A virus does not discriminate based on elections and votes.

So, what was the motivation to make the COVID-19 virus political? What was the reason for not shutting down travel? Why did Dr. Fauci ignore the early warnings that COVID-19 could possibly be a lab-created virus? We had so many questions and no real answers.

When doctors find themselves in situations like this, we usually begin by contacting other physicians from around the world. Some are friends, some are associates, and others are professionals whom we do not even know. We will also read any and all medical briefs from the WHO and CDC, looking for any bit of information that may provide a clue about the symptoms being reported and what treatment is working. Like you, we were also listening to our leaders and Dr. Anthony S. Fauci, the director of the U.S. National Institute of Allergy and Infectious Disease.

Dr. Fauci was also the Chief Medical Advisor to then-President of the United States, Donald Trump. There was also Deborah Leah Birx, who (at the time) was a physician and diplomat who served as the White House Coronavirus Response Coordinator under President Trump from 2020-2021. Dr. Fauci and Dr. Birx spoke daily, often repeatedly, throughout the day.

However, the information they provided did not make much sense to many of us. The treatment and virus-controlling strategies they provided changed rapidly.

FROM DR. TYSON: RETURNING TO EMERGENCY PREPAREDNESS PRINCIPLES

At this point, I realized I needed to use the education I had received from Loma Linda University. I had earned a Bachelor of Science in Emergency Medical Care, and part of that training was Emergency Response Preparedness. I knew we needed to have a plan in place on how we would take care of the patients as they became sick in our area.

Knowing we were the only urgent care facility in the Imperial Valley, I knew we would be busy. Safety was our first concern. Evaluation and treatment were the next priorities. We also had to worry about our family members and kids. We had staff concerns and their families to think of as well. "What would happen if someone got sick?" we asked. "What happens if I get sick, or my wife?" This was the scariest moment I have ever had as a doctor during all my years of practice.

The ODA loop was what I remembered from my training: OBSERVE what was going on, collect DATA on the event, and ACT according to that data. Then close the loop by OBSERVING the result of that action.

COVID-19 is part of the coronavirus family, I realized. I recalled we had seen a SARS outbreak (severe acute respiratory syndrome) in 2003, and it was a respiratory virus that appeared to be very dangerous at that time. This meant we needed to prepare for something likely transmitted via droplet or aerosol.

We saw the first patients coming in and began to use the protocol as planned. What we never expected were the chest X-ray findings. We noticed the radiographs revealed a patchy consolidation pattern, while the lungs themselves remained clear. This told me it was not consolidation, but more likely interstitial or inflammation causing the changes.

We discussed how we normally treated asthma patients with Solu-Medrol, a methylprednisolone or steroid, and wanted to see how it would work. We planned to give 125 milligrams of Solu-Medrol intramuscular injection to patients affected by the virus, and then revisit those patients two to three days later to recheck their chest X-rays.

While treating our patients at the urgent care center, we continued to monitor and study the findings from other frontline physicians from around the country.

We later changed to dexamethasone (a glucocorticoid medication) when the dexamethasone studies showed higher benefits for hospitalized patients. This change in medication was also good for the patient due to the inherent pain accompanying Solu-Medrol injections.

Dr. Bartlett from Texas then came out with his findings on the benefits of inhaled budesonide that appeared to help tremendously in COVID patients. We added this medicine in the nebulized form with albuterol to improve oxygenation in our patients. At the time, nebulized medications (converting liquid medication to a fine spray for inhalation) in COVID-19 were not being utilized in other hospitals because of the fear of spreading the virus to healthcare workers. But this decision was extremely worrisome for asthmatics. We had multiple asthmatics show up at our urgent care center for nebulizer treatments and intravenous Solu-Medrol, due to their inability to receive treatments in the local emergency rooms.

Other findings were blood clots and heart attacks in patients presenting with severe symptoms of COVID-19. This was when we added anticoagulants, such as aspirin or apixaban, to our treatment to prevent these complications. It was not serendipitous that we came up with these successful treatments, but it stemmed from following and treating the complications, signs, and symptoms we were seeing.

Several doctors and medical professionals around the country—and even the world—have come face-to-face with how best to treat their COVID-19 patients, many relying on hydroxychloroquine, zinc, and an antibiotic—now known commonly as the HCQ cocktail.

FROM DR. TYSON: THE VIRUS HITS HOME

In March, we saw the virus all around us—and it was terrifying. My staff was scared, my wife was scared, and my parents and in-laws were scared. Some of our young staff members had newborn kids, others had younger children, and one staffer had a teenager with Down syndrome. We had no idea how drastically our lives were about to change.

In mid-March, sick patients were pouring in, but we had no tests. Public health sent us a screening tool, but it was not helpful at all to determine if patients may or may not have COVID-19. We had so many questions and unknowns. Upper respiratory infections are common in March, but what was the difference between COVID-19 symptoms and influenza?

What about travel? People live in the border town of Mexicali, with a population of 1.5 million, and a huge number of them worked in the Imperial Valley, alongside 190,000 people.

We began screening patients outside with a pop-up tent, tables, and some chairs. Medical assistants were frightened, but strong; they took vitals and histories from patients seated in their cars. They reported back to me, and we consulted with the patients outside in chairs once the registration process was completed.

But there was still had no way to effectively test for the virus. I called the hospitals, Imperial County Public Health, and the Abbott pharmaceutical representative to see if we could order the ID kits since the FDA had approved them because we had the machine already. Across the board, the answer was "no."

There was no way to find out which patients were positive, or who needed treatment. It was frustrating and scary at the same time. My wife said we should close the office until we could figure it all out. But I was not going to give up.

I called all my contacts, and out of the blue, my good friend Terrance Korran found a lab in Orange County, EqualTox Laboratory, that could provide us with the serology tests to show if IgM or IgG immunity was present.

At last, we had a tool. We also began administering chest X-rays on all patients presenting with respiratory symptoms. It was not long before it became possible to identify the COVID-19 pattern on chest x-rays using the IgM, IgG approach. We started treatment on patients, beginning with 400 milligrams of hydroxychloroquine by mouth twice a day on the first day, then 200 milligrams three times a day for days two through five. After two to three days, patients were re-evaluated, and they would return between seven and fourteen days to ensure they improved. We also wanted to confirm immunity for patients who needed to return to work.

By the end of March and April, we were seeing 200-400 patients a day. Many essential workers asked for assistance in keeping their services and businesses open, too. We took care of the many local agencies, including the U.S. Border Patrol, Calipatria, and Centinela State Prison's corrections officers, the Department of Homeland Security, U.S. Customs, the county Sheriff's Office, the One World Beef Plant, local manufacturing businesses, multiple automobile dealerships, school districts, and Imperial County employees. Many cattle feed and farming seed companies' employees sought us out, as well as various medical and dental offices that needed to stay open.

Our system was not perfect, but it was the only one we had at the time. By revising the tents and tables inside an insulated carport with mobile clinical functions implemented, it was possible to enable air conditioning during the summer. Between providing air conditioning and essential airflow, it was possible to keep copy machines, registration kiosks, and disinfection protocols humming along on a regular basis.

There was still no concrete method to confirm patients with nose swab PCR (polymerase chain reaction) testing, due to a lack of supplies. We didn't even have personal protective equipment for our own staff members.

During this, I was contacted by the Imperial County Public Health Office. They asked me to stop testing because we were creating too much work for them, and we could not confirm our patients' infections. When I asked where else we could send them for confirmation, I was told to send patients to the emergency room.

And yet, as Gary had recounted, the problem was that in the early stages, patients were told they were not sick enough to be tested. I was informed by the emergency rooms that they only had ten swabs per week from each hospital, and only patients sent to the intensive care units were being tested.

Then I received a letter from the ER medical director at El Centro Regional Medical Center instructing me to stop prescribing hydroxychloroquine because it would prohibit the hospitals from procuring it for those who needed it. I could not believe what I was hearing. For the first time in my life as a physician, I was being told to stop saving people's lives!

My response was clear, "Give me an alternative, and I will use it. Until then, I will use whatever I have that has been shown to work."

I have never understood the pushback on using treatments that were perhaps controversial but showed promise over the ridiculous policy of "home quarantine for fourteen days" without any treatment.

Who does that? Since when is any disease treated by quarantine alone?

We have drugs that work, as well as vitamins and supplements that help; why not at least use those? Why confine others at home with known sick people? These are still questions no one in the public health department wants to answer. We went to the meetings held by public health departments and asked about the PPE (personal protective equipment) stockpile and were, once again, told nothing was available.

During this time, my staff and I were venturing out to large businesses, giving lectures on the virus and how to prevent transmission, and educating people so they understood that this treatment seemed to be working if they got sick. This information seemed to set the standard for our community: cleaning and disinfecting, social distancing, staying home when not working, and not going to work while sick. We stressed and advised early evaluation if symptoms occurred, followed by a mandatory seven days off and retesting if the serology test was negative. We also advised a mandatory fourteen days off if tests came back positive.

By May, there were two labs available to process the PCR nasal swabs. That was good and bad: while we could finally confirm cases, the level of work it took to call all the patients and get the test results out and make the follow-up and treatment calls was virtually impossible. I knew all along that the possibility of getting in trouble was there, too, so we had been keeping a spreadsheet with all the information on positive patients, our treatments, and the recovery plans.

It was good we kept those records, because when the State and CDC called in June, after months of being left alone, we learned that our center was the only place maintaining that level of detailed records. As a result, we were chosen to be the Sentinel Site for California and CDC for the Imperial Valley. It was solid validation that everything—all our record-keeping, all our treatments and protocols—were worth it.

Yet, even amid such validation, powerful forces were mobilizing, and they were prepared to do everything in their power to suppress the success we were having with our patients. The pushback was already challenging, but by June, completely unethical and dishonest information escalated the degree of resistance we faced. That information came from none other than another doctor: Dr. Mandeep Mehra, medical director of the Brigham and Women's Hospital Heart and Vascular Center and editor-in-chief of The Journal of Heart and Lung Transplantation.

CHAPTER 3

SUCCESS . . . AND THEN THE OPPOSITION BEGINS

(May – June 2020)

As the pandemic raged on throughout the spring and into the summer, the world learned more and more each day about COVID-19. First and foremost, contrary to what we were first told, this was not a natural evolution of the coronavirus from animal species into humans—making the opposition we faced completely unethical (and possibly criminal). It's unconscionable that early treatment was not being offered for something that was actually a "super" virus: genetically enhanced in a laboratory and made much more likely to be extraordinarily dangerous for humans.

Then, in May of 2020, a beacon of light shone through the darkness, in the form of a very well-written article in the *American Journal of Epidemiology* by Dr. Harvey Risch from Yale University.[1] He supported

---

1   (n.d.). Retrieved from https://academic.oup.com/aje/article/189/11/1218/5847586

early treatment with hydroxychloroquine to stem the growing numbers of hospitalizations and fatalities from COVID-19. There were 50,000-60,000 fatalities at that time, and Harvey Risch predicted there might be 100,000 dead by the end of June if this protocol was not initiated. In his Senate testimony, Dr. Risch stated, "What I have observed is that while there have been positive reports about a number of drugs, every student of outpatient use of one drug, hydroxychloroquine, with or without accompanying agents, has shown substantial benefit in reducing risks of hospitalization and mortality."[2]

Despite the success of the HCQ treatment protocol, and despite the 100% success rate for our patients who were treated early, the unthinkable happened: the NIH, FDA, WHO, and CDC knowingly blocked effective early treatment for a virus enhanced in a lab to infect and kill humans.

The reason?

To sell a vaccine that turned out to be significantly ineffective in blocking new infections by variants and gain control of the populus.

If you're wondering why the development of a vaccine has anything to do with the HCQ treatment, then it's important to know a few important details about Emergency Use Authorizations (EUAs). The COVID vaccines were allowed to be administered because they were given an EUA. However, according to the FDA, an EUA may only be granted if there is "no adequate, approved, and available alternative to the candidate product for diagnosing, preventing, or treating the disease or condition." In other words, an EUA is possible only if there is *no* other safe, effective treatment.

---

2   https://www.hsgac.senate.gov/imo/media/doc/Testimony-Risch-2020-11-19.pdf

Therefore, HCQ—and later ivermectin—had to be defeated. And the powers that be decided to take a two-pronged approach in their attack on a viable treatment:

1. Show that the protocol is dangerous. One study, published in *The Lancet* by Dr. Mandeep R. Mehra (that you will read about later in this chapter) used faulty data to create the illusion that HCQ caused cardiotoxicity (damage to the heart). However, HCQ has been used for over fifty years to effectively treat malaria—providing more than ample evidence that this drug is safe.

2. Show that the treatment is ineffective. The mainstream medical community waged this attack on the HCQ protocol in a study that not only used results from patients who were treated *late* (outside of the five-to-seven day window) but also did not use *all* of the cocktail's ingredients. Making matters worse, this particular study did not properly stratify (sort) the data, making the results and conclusions even more faulty and convoluted.[3]

One other important point is that some doctors—including Dr. Anthony Fauci—claimed that, for the studies to be deemed "sound," there needed to be a randomized control trial (RCT). This is simply statistics-speak for a research study that randomly selects certain participants in the study to receive one treatment, while another randomly-selected group receives a different treatment (or sometimes, no treatment).

3   Ladapo, J. A., McKinnon, J. E., McCullough, P. A., & Risch, H. A. (2020, January 01). "Randomized Controlled Trials of Early Ambulatory Hydroxychloroquine in the Prevention of COVID-19 Infection, Hospitalization, and Death: Meta-Analysis." Retrieved from https://www.medrxiv.org/content/10.1101/2020.09.30.20204693v1

This is yet another attempt at smoke and mirrors since a well-respected doctor (Dr. Thomas Frieden, the previous head of the CDC) published a scholarly article in *The New England Journal of Medicine* that debunks the idea that medical decisions can only be made after considering an RCT. The mainstream media has echoed similar sentiments as well, while Dr. Frieden argues that other valid data sources can be used to make critical medical decisions.

As a result of this coordinated misinformation campaign, far too many physicians were severely tainted by the misinformation campaign being waged against HCQ. They were determined to follow the NIH/CDC's guidelines of the "no early treatment approach," without any appreciation for the ability to stem COVID-19 by stopping the multiplication early in the infectious process.

This assault against scientific facts continued for months. Even today, there is little to no support or encouragement for primary doctors, emergency room doctors, or frontline doctors in general.

Fortunately, monoclonal antibodies that do neutralize COVID-19 have received EUAs to be given early via infusions or injections subcutaneously in infusion centers or ERs to help significantly since December 2020. We do recommend them widely along with the oral HCQ/IVM cocktail for best results in the prevention of hospitalization. The policy in 2020 was to do nothing other than watch patients go home and deteriorate to the point of requiring hospitalization and admission to intensive care units that require emergency life support, intubation, and mechanical ventilation. During the major pandemic surges throughout 2020, patients following this protocol had a 24% or higher likelihood of dying.

Our hospital systems were pushed to the breaking point, which should never have happened. It all could have been prevented if the

COVID-19 infections had been curtailed early in the first phase of the illness with readily available, inexpensive, and effective treatment. The massive spread of the virus would have been significantly reduced to the point where vaccines would never have been needed.

It's clear that throughout this pandemic, we've been dealing with agencies and leaders outside of the circle of empathy for compassion and consideration of the suffering, agony, and despair suffered by the millions infected with COVID-19.

Accountability is essential for the millions who suffered and died due to these blunders and crimes against humanity. Unfortunately, the conspiracy against early treatment with HCQ continued in May 2020 when academic institutions with professors like Dr. Mandeep Mehra, a cardiologist at Harvard Medical School, who published fabricated, falsified data impugning the safety and efficacy of HCQ.[4] As mentioned earlier in this chapter, Dr. Mehra attempted to make the case that HCQ could damage the heart (cardiotoxicity). Remember, this type of "data" aligned perfectly with the mainstream medical community's intention to "prove" that HCQ was dangerous, despite its use for decades in treating malaria.

And although this harmful, dishonest, and despicable travesty of science was quietly retracted in June 2020, Dr. Mehra and other conspirators went unpunished. Enormous damage had been done, creating a level of skepticism amongst the general public, thanks to the false data and the multitudes of doctors and academic institutions that perpetuated the fear and advised against the use of HCQ as an early treatment for COVID-19 infections.

---

4   (n.d.). Retrieved from https://www.thelancet.com/journals/lancet/article/PIIS0140-6736(20)31180-6/fulltext

Too many people like Drs. Fauci and Mehra—along with others on the COVID-19 task force—stood outside the circle of empathy. Without firsthand experience among real people who were suffering and dying under the scourge of COVID-19, these powerful individuals and institutions blithely accepted the casualties as collateral damage.

The most important account of the undermining of HCQ for the cure of COVID-19 was observed from within the Trump administration in March and April 2020 by Dr. Steven Hatfill. He fought against the unconscionable actions of Rick Bright and Janet Woodcock that administratively blocked HCQ and formally published and communicated on the travesty in the fall of 2021.[5]

No matter how much opposition we faced, we weren't going to give up. In fact, our own little ray of hope emerged, thanks to Pastor Richard Moore of Trinity Baptist Church of Imperial Valley, CA, a brave man who shared his healing testimony from the pulpit. In turn, this benefitted his faithful congregation, as any member who listened and trusted in the efficacy of HCQ was able to make a full recovery if they contracted this deadly virus.

But don't take our word for it. Here is Pastor Moore's Testimony:

On May 28, 2020, I was preaching to our Spanish congregation when I began to sweat profusely and ache all over my body, in my joints, and in my head and throat. The thought came to me that I had COVID-19, so as quickly as possible, I finished my message and drove home where I told my wife.

That night and the next day, I slept and felt worse with each passing hour. On May 30th, my wife took me to a clinic to be tested for COVID, and in the providence of God, I was tested by a doctor that I had recently met at a conference. He administered

5   https://www.jpands.org/vol26no3/hatfill.pdf

the test Saturday morning and called me Sunday evening to confirm my suspicions: I had COVID-19.

This doctor also prescribed hydroxychloroquine, azithromycin, and baby aspirin. For thirteen straight days, I had a fever over 100 degrees Fahrenheit, often rising above 103 degrees. I lost more than twenty pounds. It took over five weeks for me to recover, and I was unable to preach at my church until July 5th, 2020. I experienced most of the symptoms of the virus, and it took months for me to completely recover.

My wife had also contracted COVID and was sick for about nine weeks with the intestinal variety. Because of what we went through, I wanted to know how to help my church members, family members, and friends to not suffer what I went through.

I met Dr. George Fareed many years ago, as he volunteered to serve in a Medical Missions Outreach we participated in twice a year in Puerto Escondido, Mexico. Over the course of many trips, I came to know him as a highly knowledgeable doctor. I also learned he had a very compassionate heart.

Arturo Selwick, a pharmacist from Calexico, commented to me on one trip that Dr. Fareed was the smartest man he knew. Arturo was approximately ninety years old at the time he volunteered for the mission trip, so I am sure he had met a lot of intelligent people in his life. I also knew Dr. Fareed had come to the Imperial Valley to make a difference in our rural county. When I found out he was using a cocktail in his practice that was proving to be extremely effective, I reached out to him for help. I believe God used him to aid in my healing. Because of him, I added zinc to the meds I was taking, and it helped me begin to breathe better. He and Dr. Brian Tyson were advocating a treatment that used a cocktail of medicines that worked very well if given early in the onset of the virus.

Because of our friendship, my confidence in him as a doctor, and because he worked with us on missions in Mexico, I invited Dr. Fareed to come to our church to share the success that he and Dr. Tyson were having with this treatment regimen. Our people were thrilled to hear there was a treatment available that kept people from intubation and, ultimately, death.

When Dr. Fareed spoke at our church, he said if anyone gets COVID, or knew someone who had tested positive, he would be willing to prescribe them the protocol of drugs used by him and Dr. Tyson. I took the doctor at his word, and sure enough, when our church family was hit hard during a spike of COVID cases in the Imperial Valley, he prescribed the cocktail for over eighty of our members and their families.

Even though many were incredibly sick before they received the cocktail, all responded well to the treatment. Of the initial eighty, none died. Not a single person had to be intubated. At the same time, unfortunately, several of our members who hadn't heard about the cocktail ended up being hospitalized and intubated. Tragically, five of their family members died. Following this series of events, many people asked to use the drug cocktail. This led us to initiate a ministry to reach out to our friends, families, and acquaintances. Through Dr. Fareed's kindness, we have been able to help more than 800 people receive the drug protocol, and we thank God we have not had one death or intubation among those following his cocktail regimen.

We have also been able to assist and help provide medication to many underprivileged people and to those without insurance in both the Imperial Valley and the valley of Mexicali. Both valleys were hit hard by COVID. This aid was possible because we received thousands of dollars in donations from people who were blessed by the protocol of Dr. Tyson and Dr. Fareed.

Many donors sent funds just to help others get well, and countless patients have been healed by the meds they received due to this generosity. As soon as they began the protocol medications, they improved, and because of their improvement, they in turn donated to the COVID-19 fund we set up to enable more people to receive the necessary help. These recovered COVID patients also paid it forward to enable pastors and their families, many poor people, and people without insurance, to receive the necessary medicines.

Many times, our COVID-19 fund workers purchase the medications and deliver them directly to the homes of patients. Sometimes the pharmacies deliver. We are grateful God opened this door of ministry for our church to help people in their time of need.

We are pleased to be able to ease physical pain and suffering with the drug cocktails given out; to help spiritually, with the Word of God and prayer; and to give financially, with the money donated to our COVID-19 relief fund.

Overall, it has been a fulfilling, soul-satisfying experience to be a small part of this service. It would not have been possible without the expertise and generosity of both Dr. Tyson and Dr. Fareed.

The most difficult thing for me was witnessing the suppression of the use of early treatment and Dr. Fareed's protocol by social media, many pharmacists, other medical professionals, and even family and friends who Google and without knowledge, encourage people not to take the cocktail or follow the doctors' protocol.

There have been many times we worked hard to connect COVID patients with Dr. Fareed and then had someone keep that patient from using the cocktail. We have experienced instances of Dr. Fareed calling in the prescriptions, and then we heard that the pharmacist talked the patient out of taking the medicines, or even literally withheld part of the cocktail without advising the patient.

A few times, people have gotten sick, but when we were advised the patient's symptoms had worsened, we usually discover an essential medicine was left out of the prescription. Fortunately, as soon as the patient was given the essential medicine and used it correctly, they got well quickly.

Having personally seen such positive results from the use of the Drs. Tyson/Fareed protocol, it disheartens me to know people are told not to take the medications because of "safety issues."

Our results include hundreds of patients who took the drug cocktails—with no deaths or intubations. The only side effects we have heard about is nausea, which is also a symptom of COVID-19.

One person was reported as allergic to the antibiotic and subsequently stopped taking that one medication, but they continued with the rest of the cocktail protocol and made a speedy recovery. All of this is from my perspective as a pastor who seeks to promote healing for all my parishioners.

It was encouraging to witness dozens of pastors who took the cocktail as they recovered quickly and were able to return to their ministries. I personally know over a dozen pastors who died from COVID but were not given the drug cocktail. Most did not even know it existed or was available. I pray many will be encouraged to give early treatment a try. It works, it is safe, it eases pain, and it saves lives. It is relatively inexpensive, and if help is needed in acquiring the medicines, the COVID-19 relief fund can help with the costs.

I encourage us all to not forget the spiritual part of healing. We believe the greatest healer is Jesus Christ. We are willing to pray for you and share with you. Just give us a call.

Respectfully submitted,
Pastor Richard Moore
Trinity Baptist Church of Imperial Valley
Holtville, CA
September 2021

Note: Since this testimony was originally printed, the COVID-19 relief fund has given out 1,200 C19 cocktails to the larger community as of November 2021. And I am sure they will far exceed this number at the rate they are going. So many people have suffered less, and many give credit to the C19 cocktail and Drs. Fareed and Tyson for saving their lives.

Doctors, thanks for making a huge difference for so many people. I am praying your book will help bring about change in this amazing time in which we live. Thanks for laying down your life for others. It is a great privilege to call you my friend and to serve God together both here and in Latin America.

As you can see from Pastor Moore's letter, the members of the congregation that followed the C-19 protocol experienced quick, successful results. Sadly, some members were either talked out of the regimen, didn't receive the appropriate cocktail, and/or were unaware that this groundbreaking treatment even existed. Though we wish we could say that everyone survived, that was simply not the case. Unfortunately, several congregants didn't use the cocktail—and they paid the ultimate price with that decision and/or lack of information.

Once again, we knew we had to keep spreading the word—from Pastor Moore's church to churches throughout the area, to anyone and everyone that would listen to (and heed) our advice. To reach a larger audience, then, we drafted a letter to Congress—and to Dr. Fauci. Read on to learn more about what we said, our hard-hitting questions . . . and how those letters were received.

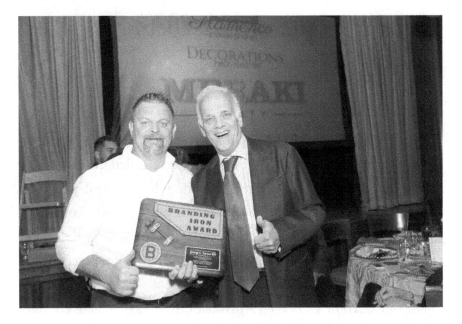

Dr. Brian Tyson (left) congratulates Dr. George Fareed for receiving the 2021 Branding Iron Award for outstanding community service during the Branding Iron Award Gala at the Stockmen's Club in Brawley, CA, September 24 (Photo credit: The Desert Review).

CHAPTER 4

LETTERS TO CONGRESS AND DR. FAUCI

(July – August 2020)

Our protocol with an HCQ backbone helped COVID-19 patients rapidly improve; in fact, the regimen has not yet failed the team since March 2020. After eight months of following this protocol, we added ivermectin to enhance the treatment. This principle was consistent with nearly thirty years of experience in treating HIV: one always employs two or three different antivirals with different mechanisms of action against HIV for successful treatment.

In our current COVID-19 protocol, there are effectively four antivirals: the main two being HCQ and ivermectin, while the secondary ones are antibiotics that have weak antiviral actions, doxycycline or azithromycin.

Zinc rounds out the protocol, as it inhibits the COVID-19 RNA-dependent polymerase. Acting intracellularly to accomplish this inhibition, zinc's entry into the cell is facilitated by HCQ, a zinc ionophore, which is a chemical species that reversibly binds ions.[6] Zinc is a positively charged metal element that needs a transporter or ionophore to pass through from the outside into the interior of living cells. Vitamin D3 also acts as a zinc ionophore, and patients with low Vitamin D levels are more vulnerable to COVID-19 infection complications. Finally, we add 325 milligrams of aspirin for protection against clotting and thrombosis (late complications of COVID-19).

Here is our most updated and successful protocol to date.[7]

The following are the drug abbreviations:

- HCQ = hydroxychloroquine
- IVM = ivermectin
- ZN = zinc sulfate
- DOXY = doxycycline
- AZM = azithromycin
- ASA = aspirin
- D3 = vitamin D3
- C19 mAbs = Eli Lilly, Glaxo or Regeneron COVID-19 monoclonal antibodies

Dosages:

- HCQ—200mg tabs #16
- ZN—22O mg (or zinc elemental 50mg) #16

---

6   Team, E.B.I.W. (n.d.). *Chebi*. Ionophore (CHEBI: 24869). Retrieved November 15, 2021, from https:// www.ebi.ac.uk/ chebi/searchld.do?chebild=24869.

7   "Local frontline doctors modify COVID treatment based on results." (2021, April 07). Retrieved from https://www. thedesertreview.com/health/local-frontline-doctors-modify-covid-treatment-based-on-results/article_9cdded9e-962f-11eb-a59a-f3e1151e98c3.html.

- DOXY—100 mg #14 or AZM- 500mg #5 or Z-pak)
- IVM—3mg tabs #12-24
- ASA—325 mg tabs #30
- D3—5,000 iu #30

Tyson/Fareed COVID-19 treatment protocols:

Day one—HCQ two tabs twice a day

- ZN capsule or tab twice a day with food
- DOXY capsule twice a day with food or AZM tab once per day
- IVM 12-18 mg on day 1, day 2, and day 3
- ASA 325mg and D3 5000 iu daily for full thirty days

Days two through five—HCQ tab three times a day

- ZN cap or tab twice a day with food
- DOXY capsule twice a day with food or AZM tab once per day
- C19 mAbs infusion from an ER/hospital or infusion center (once no later than seven days after symptoms began)
- IVM 12-18 mg on day five if symptoms warrant

If respiratory symptoms present:

- Chest x-ray and electrocardiogram, C-reactive protein, D-dimer
- Prednisone 40-60mg daily over five to seven days or dexamethasone 4 mg twice a day if oxygen saturation is less than 94% or wheezing or shortness of breath, as an oral treatment

If the patient has nebulizer access, use budesonide 0.5-1mg/2ml vía nebulizer four times a day with or without albuterol and intramuscular dexamethasone 6mg on days one and three.

- Colchicine 0.6mg twice a day over three days then 0.6mg daily over ten days
- +/- fluvoxamine 50 mg twice a day over five days
- Pepcid 20 mg daily
- Singulair 10mg at bedtime

Alternative C19 early treatment regimen:

Start if you get COVID-19

- Days one through five—HCQ tab (200 mg) twice a day for five days
- IVM 3mg tabs take 12-18 mg (5-6 tabs) by mouth daily for two days minimum and continue the same dose (12-18 mg) daily until recovered for up to a maximum of five days (take no more than five total doses of IVM)
- C19 mAbs infusion from an ER/hospital or infusion center
- Take 1 HCQ tab every week on the same day until the pandemic is over.

If respiratory symptoms increase (worsen):

- Prednisone 40-60mg daily over five to seven days or dexamethasone 4mg twice a day if oxygen saturation is less than 94% or if wheezing or shortness of breath is worsening

- Budesonide 0.5-1mg/2ml vía nebulizer two to four times a day
- Colchicine 0.6mg twice a day over three days then 0.6mg daily over ten days
- D3 5000 iu daily
- Pepcid 20 mg daily
- Montelukast (Singulair) 10mg orally daily
- Cyproheptadine (Periactin) 8mg orally three times a day
- Fenofibrate 54 mg orally three times (or 150 mg once) a day

Continue daily ASA 325mg

- Zinc 50mg daily

Armed with this powerful protocol, we pleaded throughout June and July for our representatives in the Congress and the health department to see our successful treatment—but to absolutely no avail.

FROM DR. FAREED: LETTERS TO CONGRESS & THE PRESIDENT

Considering the resistance we were facing, I penned the following letter from the Imperial Valley to California Congressman Juan Vargas and others in the state government on July 11, 2020. I sent a similar letter sent to President Donald Trump and submitted the letter below as an op-ed to a local paper, so it might be run in its entirety:

My name is Dr. George Fareed. I am a physician in Imperial County, California, which has been hit hard by the COVID-19 pandemic. I take care of patients on both an outpatient and inpatient basis, as well as nursing home patients, the most vulnerable among us.

In this letter, I am proposing a medical strategy that can help us not only through this current crisis, but also that will enable us to approach outbreaks of COVID-19 that may occur in the future.

In my attempts to keep people alive, I have had an opportunity to use many different types of treatments—remdesivir, dexamethasone, convalescent plasma replacement, etc. Yet, by far the best tool beyond supportive care with oxygen has been the combination of hydroxychloroquine (HCQ), with either azithromycin or doxycycline and zinc.

This "HCQ cocktail" (that costs less than $100) has enabled me to prevent patients from being admitted to the hospital, as well as help those patients that are hospitalized. The key is giving the HCQ cocktail early, within the first five days of the disease.

Not only have I seen outstanding results with this approach, [but I have also] not seen any patient exhibit serious side effects. To be clear—this drug has been used as an antimalarial and to treat systemic lupus erythematosus as well as rheumatoid arthritis and has over a fifty-year track record for safety. It is shocking that it is only now being characterized as a dangerous drug.

Moreover, I am in my seventies, and I (as well as some other older physicians in the hospital) use hydroxychloroquine and zinc as prophylaxis. None of us have contracted the disease despite our high exposure to COVID patients, nor have we experienced any side effects.

Despite the characterization in the mainstream media as the drug being "ineffective" and "dangerous," the evidence in the literature tells a different story. I am not only an "MD," but a former Harvard Medical School assistant professor and UCLA School of Medicine associate professor as well and am very competent at evaluating studies.

There is ample evidence now that the HCQ cocktail is effective, and there is no good evidence that there are significant side effects. Yet, like many of my colleagues in the trenches treating COVID, I find myself being obstructed on different levels from treating my patients with hydroxychloroquine.

The next option is remdesivir, which in my opinion is inferior and very expensive. Moreover, that drug is not readily available and is rationed by hospitals. Despite the representations by Dr. (Anthony) Fauci and others, there is less evidence supporting the use of Remdesivir than hydroxychloroquine.

To be clear, hydroxychloroquine is normally not helpful when given to very ill patients. Unfortunately, most of the studies have evaluated this drug only in that context. The HCQ cocktail is best used to prevent patients from getting to that dire stage. This is all so tragic because the use of HCQ cocktail would solve some of the very basic problems we are now facing:

#1   The HCQ cocktail can be used for outpatients to prevent hospitalizations and thus keep our hospitals and ICUs from being overrun with COVID patients.

#2   The HCQ cocktail can be used early on in hospitalization to prevent patients from requiring mechanical ventilation and reducing the length of hospital stay.

#3   HCQ/zinc can be used for prophylaxis for high-risk individuals including front line health providers, first responders, and even teachers who are at high risk for COVID.

As a physician, I am committed to my patients as well as doing my part to solve the COVID crisis. It has been deflating to see how the "science" has been corrupted and manipulated in an effort to disparage hydroxychloroquine. The fact that both Lancet and the New England Journal of Medicine had to retract articles relevant to hydroxychloroquine due to gross manipulation and mischaracterization of data goes to the heart of what is best characterized as a smear campaign.

As an example of the faulty science—one study (University of Minnesota) was cited in the mainstream media as disproving the effectiveness of hydroxychloroquine as "prophylaxis." Yet the patients received the drug one to four days **after** exposure. That is not prophylaxis at all—the drug must be taken **prior** to exposure. This is just one example of the non-scientific way the drug has been evaluated and the subsequent mainstream media mischaracterizations.

I am writing to you out of the frustration of knowing that there is a solution but watching as our country flounders in dealing with COVID-19. In my opinion, tens of thousands are dying unnecessarily. Our current approach of waiting for these high-risk patients to become ill and then hospitalizing them is failing.

The answer is early diagnosis of the high-risk individuals, and then treating them as outpatients with the HCQ cocktail to prevent hospitalization. So, what I am proposing is a drastic shift from our current approach: we need to ramp up our outpatient efforts of treating COVID-19 to decrease the burden on hospitals and save lives. Such an approach requires an effective outpatient treatment; we have that in the HCQ cocktail.

How do we get there? I propose a congressional hearing in which our elected representatives could listen to clinicians like myself and researchers specifically regarding the HCQ cocktail (as well as the HCQ/zinc prophylaxis treatment) and how it can help us change to a model focused on outpatient treatment and prevention, as opposed to a hospital-based approach only treating patients when they become ill.

The FDA and CDC should be there as well, given that they are the agencies that formulate the drug policies.

We need a medical strategy, not only for now while we are in a crisis, but for the future. There is no guarantee that a vaccine will rid us of COVID-19. If we had a strategy, we would not have to shut down American life, especially schools, every time there is an outbreak. We should be seeking a solution that will save as many lives as possible, and the outpatient-based approach that I and some other doctors have been advocating will best accomplish that goal.

I hope you consider my proposal, and I look forward to hearing from you.[8]

Sincerely yours,

George C. Fareed, M.D.
CMA Rural Physician of the Year 2015
Brawley, CA 92227

---

8   News, I. C., Dr. George Fareed and Richard Montenegro Brownon July 16, 2., Also, S., News, I. R., Elizabeth Varinon August 19, 2., News, I. P., . . . Julio Morales and Richard Montenegro BrownPublic SafetyRegional News. (2020, July 16). "Physician Proposes Medical Strategy Using 'HCQ'." Retrieved from https://calexicochronicle.com/2020/07/16/physician-proposes-medical-strategy-using-hcq/.

Next, we tried to convince the mainstream medical community, including Dr. Fauci, to come to their senses and do what was needed and right for our patients. It was time for them to lead the world in the *right* direction. Once again, they rebuffed our efforts. At this point, we directed our letters directly to Dr. Fauci in early August 2020. We sent a shortened version of this letter to him and the NIH:

August 12, 2020
Anthony Fauci, MD
National Institute of Allergy and Infectious Diseases
Washington, D.C.

Dear Dr. Fauci:

You were placed into the most high-profile role regarding America's response to the coronavirus pandemic. Americans have relied on your medical expertise concerning the wearing of masks, resuming employment, returning to school, and of course, medical treatment.

You are largely unchallenged in terms of your medical opinions. You are the de facto "COVID-19 Czar." This is unusual in the medical profession, in which doctors' opinions are challenged by other physicians in the form of exchanges between doctors at hospitals, medical conferences, as well as debate in medical journals. You render your opinions unchallenged, without formal public opposition from physicians who passionately disagree with you. It is incontestable that the public is best served when opinions and policy are based on the prevailing evidence and science and [are] able to withstand the scrutiny of medical professionals.

As experience accrued in treating COVID-19 infections, physicians worldwide discovered that high-risk patients can be treated successfully as an outpatient, within the first five to seven days of the onset of symptoms, with a "cocktail" consisting of hydroxychloroquine, zinc, and azithromycin (or doxycycline). Multiple scholarly contributions to the literature detail the efficacy of the hydroxychloroquine-based combination treatment.

Dr. Harvey Risch, the renowned Yale epidemiologist, published an article in May 2020 in the American Journal of Epidemiology titled, "Early Outpatient Treatment of Symptomatic, High-Risk COVID-19 Patients that Should be Ramped-Up Immediately as Key to Pandemic Crisis."[9] He further published an article in Newsweek in July 2020 for the general public,[10] expressing the same conclusions and opinions. Dr. Risch is an expert at evaluating research data and study designs, [and he has published] over 300 articles. Dr. Risch's assessment is that there is unequivocal evidence for the early and safe use of the "HCQ cocktail." If there are Q-T interval concerns, doxycycline can be substituted for azithromycin, as it has activity against RNA viruses without any cardiac effects.

Yet, you continue to reject the use of hydroxychloroquine, except in a hospital setting in the form of clinical trials, repeatedly emphasizing the lack of evidence supporting its use. Hydroxychloroquine, despite sixty-five years of use for malaria, and over forty years for lupus and rheumatoid arthritis, with a well-established safety profile, has been deemed by you and the FDA as unsafe for use in the treatment of symptomatic COVID-19 infections. Your opinions have influenced the thinking of physicians and their patients, medical boards, state and federal agencies, pharmacists, hospitals, and just about everyone involved in medical decision-making.

Indeed, your opinions impacted the health of Americans, and many aspects of our day-to-day lives, including employment and school. Those of us who prescribe hydroxychloroquine, zinc, and azithromycin/doxycycline believe fervently that early outpatient use would save tens of thousands of lives and enable our country to dramatically

---

9   Risch, H. A. (2020, May 27). "Early Outpatient Treatment of Symptomatic, High-Risk COVID-19 Patients That Should Be Ramped Up Immediately as Key to the Pandemic Crisis." Retrieved from https://academic.oup.com/aje/article/189/11/1218/5847586.

10 Harvey A. Risch, M. (2020, July 28). "The Key to Defeating COVID-19 Already Exists. We Need to Start Using It | Opinion." Retrieved from https://www.newsweek.com/key-defeating-covid-19-already-exists-we-need-start-using-it-opinion-1519535.

alter the response to COVID-19. We advocate for an approach that will reduce fear and allow Americans to get their lives back.

We hope our questions compel you to reconsider your current approach to COVID-19 infection.

QUESTIONS REGARDING EARLY OUTPATIENT TREATMENT:

1. *There are generally two stages of COVID-19 symptomatic infection: initial flu-like symptoms with progression to cytokine storm and respiratory failure, correct?*
2. *When people are admitted to a hospital, they generally are in worse condition, correct?*
3. *There are no specific medications currently recommended for early outpatient treatment of symptomatic COVID-19 infection, correct?*
4. *Remdesivir and dexamethasone are used for hospitalized patients, correct?*
5. *There is currently no recommended pharmacologic early outpatient treatment for individuals in the flu stage of the illness, correct?*
6. *It is true that COVID-19 is much more lethal than the flu for high-risk individuals such as older patients and those with significant comorbidities, correct?*
7. *Individuals with signs of early COVID-19 infection typically have a runny nose, fever, cough, shortness of breath, loss of smell, etc., and physicians send them home to rest, eat chicken soup etc., but offer no specific, targeted medications, correct?*
8. *These high-risk individuals are at high risk of death, on the order of 15 percent or higher, correct?*
9. *So just so we are clear—the current standard of care now is to send clinically stable symptomatic patients home "with a wait and see" approach?*
10. *Are you aware that physicians are successfully using hydroxychloroquine combined with zinc and azithromycin as a "cocktail" for early outpatient treatment of symptomatic, high-risk, individuals?*
11. *Have you heard of the "Zelenko Protocol" for treating high-risk patients with COVID-19 as an outpatient?*

12. *Have you read Dr. Risch's article in the American Journal of Epidemiology of the early outpatient treatment of COVID-19?*

13. *Are you aware that physicians using the medication combination or "cocktail" recommend use within the first five to seven days of the onset of symptoms, before the illness impacts the lungs, or cytokine storm evolves?*

14. *Again, to be clear, your recommendation is no pharmacologic treatment as an outpatient for the flu-like symptoms in patients that are stable, regardless of their risk factors, correct?*

15. *Would you advocate for early pharmacologic outpatient treatment of symptomatic COVID-19 patients if you were confident that it was beneficial?*

16. *Are you aware that there are hundreds of physicians in the United States and thousands across the globe who have had dramatic success treating high-risk individuals as outpatients with this "cocktail?"*

17. *Are you aware that there are at least ten studies demonstrating the efficacy of early outpatient treatment with the Hydroxychloroquine cocktail for high-risk patients—so this is beyond anecdotal, correct?*

18. *If one of your loved ones had diabetes or asthma, or any potentially complicating comorbidity, and tested positive for COVID-19, would you recommend "wait and see how they do" and [only] go to the hospital if symptoms progress?*

19. *Even with multiple studies documenting remarkable outpatient efficacy and safety of the hydroxychloroquine "cocktail," you believe the risks of the medication combination outweigh the benefits?*

20. *Is it true that with regard to hydroxychloroquine and treatment of COVID-19 infection, you have said repeatedly that "the overwhelming evidence of properly conducted randomized clinical trials indicate no therapeutic efficacy of Hydroxychloroquine (HCQ)"?*

21. *But **none** of the randomized controlled trials to which you refer were done in the first five to seven days after the onset of symptoms, correct?*

22. *All of the randomized controlled trials to which you refer were done on hospitalized patients, correct?*

23. *Hospitalized patients are typically sicker than outpatients, correct?*

24. *None of the randomized controlled trials to which you refer used the full cocktail consisting of hydroxychloroquine, zinc, and azithromycin, correct?*

25. *While the University of Minnesota study is referred to as disproving the cocktail, the meds were not given within the first five to seven days of illness, the test group was not high risk (death rates were 3 percent), and no zinc was given, correct?*

26. *Again, for clarity, the trials upon which you base your opinion regarding the efficacy of hydroxychloroquine assessed neither the full cocktail (to include zinc and azithromycin or doxycycline) nor administered treatment within the first five to seven days of symptoms, nor focused on the high-risk group, correct?*

27. *Therefore, you have no basis to conclude that the hydroxychloroquine cocktail when used early in the outpatient setting, within the first five to seven days of symptoms, in high-risk patients, is not effective, correct?*

28. *It is thus false and misleading to say that the effective and safe use of hydroxychloroquine, zinc, and azithromycin has been "debunked," correct? How could it be "debunked" if there is not a single study that contradicts its use?*

29. *Should it not be an absolute priority for the NIH and CDC to look at ways to treat Americans with symptomatic COVID-19 infections early to prevent disease progression?*

30. *The SARS-CoV-2/COVID-19 virus is an RNA virus. It is well-established that zinc interferes with RNA viral replication, correct?*

31. *Moreover, is it not true that hydroxychloroquine facilitates the entry of zinc into the cell, [as] an "ionophore," correct?*

32. *Isn't it also true that azithromycin has established anti-viral properties?*

33. *Are you aware of the paper from Baylor by Dr. McCullough et. al. describing established mechanisms by which the components of the "HCQ cocktail" exert antiviral effects?*

34. *So, the use of hydroxychloroquine, azithromycin (or doxycycline), and zinc—the "HCQ cocktail"—is based on science, correct?*

QUESTIONS REGARDING SAFETY:

1. The FDA writes the following: "In light of ongoing serious cardiac adverse events and their serious side effects, the known and potential benefits of CQ and HCQ no longer outweigh the known and potential risks for authorized use." So, not only is the FDA saying that hydroxychloroquine doesn't work, [but] they are also saying that it is a very dangerous drug. Yet, is it not true the drug has been used as an anti-malarial drug for over sixty-five years?

2. Isn't it true that the drug has been used for lupus and rheumatoid arthritis for many years at similar doses?

3. Do you know of even a single study prior to COVID-19 that has provided definitive evidence against the use of the drug based on safety concerns?

4. Are you aware that chloroquine or hydroxychloroquine has many approved uses for hydroxychloroquine, advanced neurological sarcoidosis,[11] sensitizing breast cancer cells for chemotherapy [2012 study], the attenuation of renal ischemia [2018 study], lupus nephritis [2006 study], [and] epithelial ovarian cancer [2020 study], just to name a few? Where are the cardiotoxicity concerns ever mentioned?

5. Dr. Risch estimates the risk of cardiac death from hydroxychloroquine to be 9/100,000 using the data provided by the FDA. That does not seem to be a high risk, considering the risk of death in an older patient with comorbidities can be 15 percent or more. Do you consider 9/100,000 to be a high risk when weighed against the risk of death in older patients with comorbidities?

6. To put this in perspective, the drug [has been] used for sixty-five years without warnings [aside from the need for periodic retinal checks], but the FDA somehow [felt] the need to send out an alert on June 15 that the drug is dangerous. Does that make any logical sense to you, Dr. Fauci, based on "science"?

---

11 Sharma, Om P., M.D. "Effectiveness of Chloroquine and Hydroxychloroquine in Treating Selected Patients With Sarcoidosis With Neurological Involvement." *JAMA Network*, 1988. Retrieved from https://jamanetwork.com/journals/jamaneurology/fullarticle/774209.

7. *Moreover, consider that the protocols for usage in early treatment are for five to seven days, at relatively low doses of hydroxychloroquine, similar to what is being given in other diseases (RA, SLE) over many years. Does it make any sense to you logically that a five-to-seven-day dose of hydroxychloroquine, when not given in high doses, could be considered dangerous?*

8. *You are also aware that articles published in the New England Journal of Medicine, The Lancet, and one out of Harvard University, regarding the dangers of hydroxychloroquine, had to be retracted based on the fact that the data was fabricated. Are you aware of that?*

9. *If there was such good data on the risks of hydroxychloroquine, one would not have to use fake data, correct?*

10. *After all, sixty-five years is a long-time to determine whether or not a drug is safe, do you agree?*

11. *In the clinical trials that you have referenced (e.g., the Minnesota and the Brazil studies), there was not a single death attributed directly to hydroxychloroquine, correct?*

12. *According to Dr. Risch, there is no evidence based on the data to conclude that hydroxychloroquine is a dangerous drug. Are you aware of any published report that rebuts Dr. Risch's findings?*

13. *Are you aware that the FDA ruling, along with your statements, have led Governors in a number of states to restrict the use of hydroxychloroquine?*

14. *Are you aware that pharmacies are not filling prescriptions for this medication based on your and the FDA's restrictions?*

15. *Are you aware that doctors are being punished by state medical boards for prescribing the medication based on your comments, as well as the FDA's?*

16. *Are you aware that people who want the medication sometimes need to call physicians in other states, pleading for it?*

17. *And yet, you opined in March that while people were dying at the rate of 10,000 patients a week, hydroxychloroquine could only be used in an inpatient setting as part of a clinical trial, correct?*

18. *So, people who want to be treated in that critical five-to-seven-day period and avoid being hospitalized are basically out of luck in your view, correct?*

19. *So again, for clarity, without a shred of evidence that the hydroxychloroquine/HCQ cocktail is dangerous in the doses currently recommended for early outpatient treatment, you and the FDA have made it very difficult, if not impossible in some cases, to get this treatment, correct?*

QUESTIONS REGARDING METHODOLOGY:

1. *In regard to the use of hydroxychloroquine, you have repeatedly made the same statement: "The overwhelming evidence from properly conducted randomized clinical trials indicate no therapeutic efficacy of hydroxychloroquine." Is that correct?*

2. *In Dr. Risch's article regarding the early use of hydroxychloroquine, he disputes your opinion. He scientifically evaluated the data from the studies to support his opinions. Have you published any articles to support your opinions?*

3. *You repeatedly state that randomized clinical trials are needed to make conclusions regarding treatments, correct?*

4. *The FDA has approved many medications (especially in the area of cancer treatment) without randomized clinical trials, correct?*

5. *Are you aware that Dr. Thomas Frieden, the previous head of the CDC, wrote an article in the New England Journal of Medicine in 2017: "Evidence for Health Decision Making— Beyond Randomized Clinical Trials (RCT)?" Have you read that article?*

6. *In it, Dr. Frieden states that "many data sources can provide valid evidence for clinical and public health action, including analysis of aggregate clinical or epidemiological data." Do you disagree with that?*

7. *Frieden discusses "practice-based evidence" as being essential in many discoveries, such as SIDS (sudden infant death syndrome). Do you disagree with that?*

8. *Frieden writes the following: "Current evidence-grading systems are biased toward randomized clinical trials, which may lead to inadequate consideration of non-*

RCT data." Dr. Fauci, have you considered all the non-RCT data in coming to your opinions?

9. Dr. Risch, who is a leading world authority in the analysis of aggregate clinical data, has done a rigorous analysis that he published regarding the early treatment of COVID-19 with hydroxychloroquine, zinc, and azithromycin. He cites five or six studies, and in an updated article there are five or six more. [This equates to] a total of ten to twelve clinical studies with formally collected data specifically regarding the early treatment of COVID. Have you analyzed the aggregate data regarding early treatment of high-risk patients with hydroxychloroquine, zinc, and azithromycin?

10. Is there any document that you can produce for the American people of your analysis of the aggregate data that would rebut Dr. Risch's analysis?

11. Yet, despite what Dr. Risch believes is overwhelming evidence in support of the early use of hydroxychloroquine, you dismiss the treatment insisting on randomized controlled trials, even in the midst of a pandemic?

12. Would you want a loved one with high-risk comorbidities placed in the control group of a randomized clinical trial, when a number of studies demonstrate safety and dramatic efficacy of the early use of the hydroxychloroquine "cocktail?"

13. Are you aware that the FDA approved a number of cancer chemotherapy drugs without randomized control trials, based solely on epidemiological evidence? The trials came later as confirmation. Are you aware of that?

14. You are well aware that there were no randomized clinical trials in the case of penicillin that saved thousands of lives in World War II. Was this not in the best interest of our soldiers?

15. You would agree that many lives were saved with the use of cancer drugs and penicillin that were used before any randomized clinical trials, correct?

16. You have referred to evidence for hydroxychloroquine as "anecdotal," which is defined as "evidence collected in a casual or informal manner and relying heavily or entirely on personal testimony," correct?

17. *Are you aware that there are many studies supporting the use of hydroxychloroquine in which evidence was collected formally and not on personal testimony?*

18. *So, it would be false to conclude that the evidence supporting the early use of hydroxychloroquine is anecdotal, correct?*

COMPARISON BETWEEN U.S. AND OTHER COUNTRIES REGARDING CASE FATALITY RATE:

(DR. FAUCI: IT WOULD BE VERY HELPFUL TO HAVE THE GRAPHS COMPARING OUR CASE FATALITY RATES TO OTHER COUNTRIES.)

Are you aware that countries like Senegal and Nigeria (that use hydroxychloroquine) have much lower case-fatality rates than the United States?

1. *Have you pondered the relationship between the use of hydroxychloroquine by a given country and their case mortality rate, and [have you pondered] why there is a strong correlation between the use of HCQ and the reduction of the case mortality rate?*

2. *Have you considered consulting with a country (such as India) that has had great success treating COVID-19 prophylactically?*

3. *Why shouldn't our first responders and frontline workers who are at high risk at least have an option of HCQ/zinc prophylaxis?*

4. *We should all agree that countries with far inferior healthcare delivery systems should not have lower case fatality rates. Reducing our case fatality rate from nearly 5 percent to 2.5 percent (in line with many countries who use HCQ early) would have cut our total number of deaths in half, correct?*

5. *Why not consult with countries who have lower case-fatality rates, even without expensive medicines such as remdesivir and far less advanced intensive care capabilities?*

GIVING AMERICANS THE OPTION TO USE HCQ FOR COVID-19:

1. *Harvey Risch, the pre-eminent epidemiologist from Yale, wrote a Newsweek article titled: "The Key to Defeating COVID-19 Already Exists. We Need to Start Using It."[12] Did you read the article?*

2. *Are you aware that the cost of the hydroxychloroquine "cocktail," including the Z-pack and zinc, is about $50?*

3. *Are you aware the cost of remdesivir is about $3,200?*

4. *So that's about sixty doses of the HCQ "cocktail," correct?*

5. *In fact, President Trump had the foresight to amass sixty million doses of hydroxychloroquine, and yet you continue to stand in the way of doctors who want to use that medication for their infected patients, correct?*

6. *Those are a lot of doses of medication that potentially could be used to treat our poor, especially our minority populations and people of color that have a difficult time accessing healthcare. They die more frequently of COVID-19, do they not?*

7. *But because of your obstinance blocking the use of HCQ, this stockpile has remained largely unused, correct?*

8. *Would you acknowledge that your strategy of telling Americans to restrict their behavior, wear masks, and distance, and put their lives on hold indefinitely until there is a vaccine is not working?*

9. *So, 160,000 deaths later, [with] an economy in shambles, kids out of school, suicides and drug overdoses at a record high, people neglected and dying from other medical conditions, and America reacting to every outbreak with another lockdown—is it not time to re-think your strategy that is fully dependent on an effective vaccine?*

10. *Why not consider a strategy that protects the most vulnerable and allows Americans back to living their lives and not wait for a vaccine panacea that may never come?*

12 Harvey A. Risch, M. (2020, July 28). "The Key to Defeating COVID-19 Already Exists. We Need to Start Using It | Opinion." Retrieved from https://www.newsweek.com/key-defeating-covid-19-already-exists-we-need-start-using-it-opinion-1519535.

11. *Why not consider the approach that thousands of doctors around the world are using, supported by a number of studies in the literature, with early outpatient treatment of high-risk patients for typically one week with HCQ, zinc, and azithromycin?*

12. *You don't see a problem with the fact that the government, due to your position, in some cases interferes with the choice of using HCQ? Should not that be a choice between the doctor and the patient?*

13. *While some doctors may not want to use the drug, should not doctors who believe that it is indicated be able to offer it to their patients?*

14. *Are you aware that doctors who are publicly advocating for such a strategy with the early use of the HCQ cocktail are being silenced with the removal of content on the internet and even censorship in the medical community?*

15. *You are aware of the twenty or so physicians who came to the Supreme Court steps advocating for the early use of the hydroxychloroquine cocktail. In fact, you said these were "a bunch of people spouting out something that isn't true." Dr. Fauci, these are not just "people"; these are doctors who actually treat patients—unlike you, correct?*

16. *Do you know that the video they made went viral with seventeen million views in just a few hours—and was then removed from the internet?*

17. *Are you aware that their website, American Frontline Doctors, was taken down the next day?*

18. *Did you see the way that Nigerian immigrant physician, Dr. Stella Immanuel, was mocked in the media for her religious views and called a "witch doctor"?*

19. *Are you aware that Dr. Simone Gold, the leader of the group, was fired from her job as an emergency room physician the following day?*

20. *Are you aware that physicians advocating for this treatment, which has by now probably saved millions of lives around the globe, are harassed by local health departments, state agencies and medical boards, and even at their own hospitals? Are you aware of that?*

21. *Don't you think doctors should have the right to speak out on behalf of their patients without the threat of retribution?*

22. *Are you aware that videos and other educational information are removed off the internet and labeled, in the words of Mark Zuckerberg, as "misinformation"?*

23. *Is it not misinformation to characterize hydroxychloroquine, in the doses used for early outpatient treatment of COVID-19 infections, as a dangerous drug?*

24. *Is it not misleading for you to repeatedly state to the American public that randomized clinical trials are the sole source of information to confirm the efficacy of a treatment?*

25. *Was it not misinformation when on CNN you cited the Lancet study based on false data from Surgisphere as evidence of the lack of efficacy of hydroxychloroquine?*

26. *As a result of your comments repeated in the MSM, is it not misinformation that a randomized clinical trial is required by the FDA for a drug approval?*

27. *Don't you realize how much damage this falsehood perpetuates?*

28. *How is it not misinformation for you and the FDA to keep telling the American public that hydroxychloroquine is dangerous when you know that there is nothing more than anecdotal evidence of that?*

29. *Dr. Fauci, if you or a loved one were infected with COVID-19 and had flu-like symptoms, and you knew as you do now, that there is a safe and effective cocktail that you could take to prevent worsening and the possibility of hospitalization, can you honestly tell us that you would refuse the medication?*

30. *Why not give our healthcare workers and first responders, who even with the necessary PPE are contracting the virus at a three to four times greater rate than the general public, the right to choose (along with their doctor) if they want to use the medicine prophylactically?*

31. *Why is the government inserting itself in a way that is unprecedented in regard to a historically safe medication and not allowing patients the right to choose, along with their doctor?*

32. *Why not give the American people the right to decide (along with their physician) whether or not they want outpatient treatment in the first five to seven days of the disease with a cocktail that is safe and costs around fifty dollars?*

FINAL QUESTIONS:

1. Dr. Fauci, please explain how a randomized clinical trial, to which you repeatedly make reference, for testing the HCQ cocktail (hydroxychloroquine, azithromycin, and zinc) administered within five to seven days of the onset of symptoms is even possible now given the declining case numbers in so many states?

2. For example, if the NIH were now to direct a study to begin September 15, where would such a study be done?

3. Please explain how a randomized study on the early treatment (within the first five to seven days of symptoms) of high-risk, symptomatic COVID-19 infections could be done during the influenza season and be valid?

4. Please explain how multiple observational studies arrive at the same outcomes using the same formulation of hydroxychloroquine, azithromycin, and zinc, given in the same timeframe for the same study population (high-risk patients), is not evidence that the cocktail works?

5. In fact, how is it not significant evidence, during a pandemic, for hundreds of non-academic private practice physicians to achieve the same outcomes with the early use of the HCQ cocktail?

6. What is your recommendation for the medical management of a seventy-five-year-old diabetic with fever, cough, and loss of smell, but not yet hypoxic, whom emergency room providers do not feel warrants admission? We know that hundreds of U.S. physicians (and thousands more around the world) would manage this case with the HCQ cocktail with predictable success.

7. If you were in charge in 1940, would you have advised the mass production of penicillin based primarily on lab evidence and one case series on five patients in England, or would you have stated that a randomized clinical trial was needed?

8. Why would any physician put their medical license, professional reputation, and job on the line to recommend the HCQ cocktail—that does not make them any money—unless they knew the treatment could significantly help their patient?

9. Why would a physician take the medication themselves and prescribe it to family members (for treatment or prophylaxis) unless they felt strongly that the medication was beneficial?

10. How is it informed and ethical medical practice to allow a COVID-19 patient to deteriorate in the early stages of the infection when there is an inexpensive, safe, and dramatically effective treatment with the HCQ cocktail, which the science indicates interferes with coronavirus replication?

11. How is your approach to "wait and see" in the early stages of COVID-19 infection, especially in high-risk patients, following the science?

While previous questions are related to hydroxychloroquine-based treatment, we have two questions addressing masks:

1. As you recall, you stated on March 8, just a few weeks before the devastation in the Northeast, that masks weren't needed. You later said that you made this statement to prevent a hoarding of masks that would disrupt availability to healthcare workers. Why did you not make a recommendation for people to wear any face covering to protect themselves, as we are doing now?

2. Rather, you issued no such warning, and people were riding in subways and visiting their relatives in nursing homes without any face covering. Currently, your position is that face coverings are essential. Please explain whether or not you made a mistake in early March, and how you would go about it differently now.

CONCLUSION:

Since the start of the pandemic, physicians have used hydroxychloroquine to treat symptomatic COVID-19 infections, as well as for prophylaxis. Initial results were mixed as indications and doses were explored to maximize outcomes and minimize risks. What emerged was that hydroxychloroquine appeared to work best when coupled with *azithromycin. In fact, it was the president of the United States who recommended to you publicly at the beginning of the pandemic, in early March, that you should consider early treatment with hydroxychloroquine and a "Z-pack." Additional studies showed that patients did not seem to benefit when COVID-19 infections were treated with hydroxychloroquine late in the course of the illness, typically in a hospital setting, but treatment was consistently effective, even in high-risk patients, when hydroxychloroquine was given in a "cocktail" with azithromycin and, critically, zinc in the first five to seven days after the onset of symptoms. The outcomes are, in fact, dramatic.*

As clearly presented in the McCullough article from Baylor, and described by Dr. Vladimir Zelenko, the efficacy of the HCQ cocktail is based on the pharmacology of the hydroxychloroquine ionophore acting as the "gun" and zinc as the "bullet," while azithromycin potentiates the anti-viral effect. Undeniably, the hydroxychloroquine combination treatment is supported by science. Yet, you continue to ignore the "science" behind the disease. Viral replication occurs rapidly in the first five to seven days of symptoms and can be treated at that point with the HCQ cocktail. Rather, your actions have denied patients treatment in that early stage. Without such treatment, some patients, especially those at high risk with co-morbidities, deteriorate and require hospitalization for evolving cytokine storm resulting in pneumonia, respiratory failure, and intubation with 50 percent mortality. Dismissal of the science results in bad medicine, and the outcome is over 160,000 dead Americans. Countries that have followed the science and treated the disease in the early stages have far better results, a fact that has been concealed from the American public.

Despite mounting evidence and impassioned pleas from hundreds of frontline physicians, your position was and continues to be that randomized controlled trials (RCTs) have not shown there to be a benefit. However, not a single randomized control trial has tested what is being recommended: the use of the full cocktail (especially zinc) in high-risk patients, initiated within the first five to seven days of the onset of symptoms. Using hydroxychloroquine and azithromycin late in the disease process, with or without zinc, does not produce the same, unequivocally positive results.

Dr. Thomas Frieden, in a 2017 New England Journal of Medicine article regarding randomized clinical trials, emphasized there are situations in which it is entirely appropriate to use other forms of evidence to scientifically validate a treatment. Such is the case during a pandemic that moves like a brushfire, jumping to different parts of the country. Insisting on randomized clinical trials in the midst of a pandemic is simply foolish. Dr. Harvey Risch, a world-renowned Yale epidemiologist, analyzed all the data regarding the use of the hydroxychloroquine/HCQ cocktail and concluded that the evidence of its efficacy when used early in COVID-19 infection is unequivocal.

Curiously, despite a safety record of over sixty-five years, the FDA suddenly deemed hydroxychloroquine a dangerous drug, especially with regard to cardiotoxicity. Dr. Risch analyzed data provided by the FDA and concluded that the risk of a significant cardiac event from hydroxychloroquine is extremely low, especially when compared to the mortality rate of COVID-19 patients with high-risk comorbidities. How do you reconcile that, for forty years, rheumatoid arthritis and lupus patients have been treated over long periods, often for years, with hydroxychloroquine—and now there are suddenly concerns about a five-to-seven-day course of hydroxychloroquine at similar or slightly increased doses?

The FDA statement regarding hydroxychloroquine and cardiac risk is patently false and alarmingly misleading to physicians, pharmacists, patients, and other health professionals. The benefits of the early use of hydroxychloroquine to prevent hospitalization in high-risk patients with COVID-19 infection far outweigh the risks. Physicians are not able to obtain the medication for their patients, and in some cases are restricted by their state from prescribing hydroxychloroquine. The government's obstruction of the early treatment of symptomatic high-risk COVID-19 patients with hydroxychloroquine, a medication used extensively and safely for so long, is unprecedented.

It is essential that you tell the truth to the American public regarding the safety and efficacy of the hydroxychloroquine/HCQ cocktail. The government must protect and facilitate the sacred and revered physician-patient relationship by permitting physicians to treat their patients. Governmental obfuscation and obstruction are as lethal as a cytokine storm.

Americans must not continue to die unnecessarily. Adults must resume employment and our youth [must] return to school. Locking down America while awaiting an imperfect vaccine has done far more damage to Americans than the coronavirus. We are confident that thousands of lives would be saved with early treatment of high-risk individuals with a cocktail of hydroxychloroquine, zinc, and azithromycin. Americans must not live in fear. As Dr. Harvey Risch's Newsweek article declares, "The key to defeating COVID-19 already exists. We need to start using it."

George C. Fareed, MD—Brawley, California
Michael M. Jacobs, MD, MPH—Pensacola, Florida
Donald C. Pompan, MD – Salinas, California

We never received a response from Dr. Fauci—as thousands upon thousands more people continued to die, without the potentially life-saving early treatment HCQ protocol. Why would anyone argue with the success we were experiencing? One word: money.

As you will see in the next chapter, Big Pharma doesn't really care all that much about your health. Their true priority is their bottom line. And when it came to COVID, Big Pharma, and greed, we didn't stand a chance.

CHAPTER 5
BIG PHARMA AND GREED
(Fall 2020 – January 2021)

Getting the word out about the HCQ protocol was like paddling upstream—so we tried a different route at the grassroots level. Certainly, people were hungry for this information; we just needed to find them. Knowing how confused parents and educators in our community were about returning to in-person learning during a pandemic, a school board meeting would be the perfect forum to educate and clear up people's misconceptions about our powerful early treatment option.

The following is an article published by a local Imperial Valley newspaper resulting from our efforts to share valuable information at a Brawley Board of Education meeting, in reference to students and teachers returning to school:

Dr. George Fareed, a family medicine physician with privileges at both Pioneers Memorial Healthcare District and El Centro Regional Medical Center, spoke to the Brawley Elementary School District Board of Trustees Tuesday evening, October 13, 2020, about COVID-19 and ways staff could feel safe coming back to work when schools reopen.

Fareed gave the board general information on a low dose, early treatment of hydroxychloroquine as a prophylaxis for COVID-19 that, according to him, is very safe.

"My position now is that teachers should know they can be treated, parents should know they can be treated, and they need to be encouraged and given confidence to avoid the fear that we have presented within the past at this stage," said Fareed.

According to Fareed, there is a new peer reviewed algorithm that shows hydroxychloroquine, when used in early stages, can fight back against the virus. Fareed said zinc and other healthy supplements can also be used to combat the virus by blunting its effect. Fareed said anyone can visit his office for a consultation on the treatment, saying teachers have already visited him about it.

Fareed suggested the district begin reopening and letting employees know the cocktail is an option to protect against the virus. Fareed suggested encouraging teachers to begin taking the regimen to prevent COVID, saying they respond well to the treatment and from there the parents should be encouraged as well.

He acknowledged the treatment has been labeled as dangerous, but said it is a false label.

However, Brawley Elementary Teachers Association (BETA) President Mary-Ann Moreno disagreed. Moreno said she respected Fareed as a doctor but felt the teachers should not have to take that risk.

"Why am I going to take that risk? Why are my teachers going to take that risk? When we have just gotten into the groove of distance learning and we want to reopen again?" said Moreno, "Do we really take our life for granted like that?"

Moreno said she has already lost two family members to COVID and has been unable to mourn or have a proper service for them.

She said it is an experience she would never wish any of the BESD teachers or anyone else to go through.

BESD has lost one staff member to COVID-19, something that Moreno said the district seems to have already forgotten.

California School Employees Association (CSEA) Brawley Chapter President Alejandra Rodarte echoed some of Moreno's sentiments. Rodarte said there is real fear that employees, including herself, will bring COVID home to their families if they have to return to campus.

"I feel like, as a classified employee, it's scary," said Rodarte about going back to campus. "I think it's something that would be very stressful for myself and for other employees. I have members right now who are scared to come back, or they are already at work and they are stressed all the time because they are scared to take it home."

Rodarte is concerned that even if the school sites do everything possible to keep employees and students safe, there will still be children who do not follow the rules or households that do not follow the guidelines, leaving the potential for spread, despite all safety precautions. Rodarte questioned if there would be enough of Fareed's cocktail to go around, especially if other Imperial Valley schools reopen.

Both Moreno and Rodarte said BESD would have to meet county requirements and guidelines before the campuses should consider reopening. Even then, the district would have to meet with the staff and labor representatives before considering moving into a hybrid, on-campus learning curriculum, despite what Fareed suggests.[13]

---

13 Ramos, K. (2020, November 23). "Dr. Fareed speaks COVID treatment with BESD." Retrieved from https://www.thedesertreview.com/education/dr-fareed-speaks-covid-treatment-with-besd/article_d4217e16-11ea-11eb-853a-a754030db598.html.

While our attendance at this board meeting was well-received by some people who were present, we were still fighting the overwhelming fear of many staff members. To be honest, this was understandable, given the mass messaging they were hearing in the mainstream media. But we soldiered on, determined to elevate our message and take on even more challenging audiences, filled with opponents whose insatiable greed— both politically and economically—were distorting and skewing all communication, from media messaging to medical education.

Medical education has been negligent in publicizing the efficacies and safety of repurposed, generic, multifunctional agents. This enormous compromise results in human suffering and death in return for huge profits, riches, and power for pharmaceutical companies and anyone with a financial interest in this area—despite economic ruin for the majority of Americans.

In the fall of 2020, Senator Ron Johnson and his staff in Washington called for a Senate hearing on the Early Treatment of COVID-19. Dr. Fareed was one of three physician witnesses to testify under oath to the Homeland Security Committee of the U.S. Senate on November 19, 2020. Dr. Peter McCullough from Texas A&M and Baylor University Medical Center, and Dr. Harvey Risch from Yale University, were the other witnesses for the Republican majority.

During his testimony, with great trepidation and respect, Fareed stated the following:

I have a background in virology from a research standpoint from work at the NIAID (NIH) and as a professor performing research at Harvard Medical School (after I graduated from Harvard Medical School in 1970, I became a professor there) and at UCLA School of Medicine. I have had thirty years of clinical experience, treating HIV and other infectious diseases, as well as practicing primary care medicine.

I have experience treating COVID patients both in the flu stage as outpatients, but also as hospitalized inpatients—even in the ICU.

Like everything else in medicine, the goal is to treat early; COVID patients are difficult to treat when they get very sick.

The Imperial Valley, where I work, became the COVID epicenter for California in June and July of 2020. Since early March, both in my Brawley clinic and Dr. Brian Tyson's All Valley Urgent Care Clinic in El Centro (where I also work), over 25,000 fearful people were screened, over 2,400 were COVID-19 positive, and we successfully treated hundreds of the high risk and symptomatic ones.

We have always used a triple HCQ cocktail; HCQ (3200 milligrams, over five days), azithromycin or doxycycline, and especially zinc, which is often left out in the studies. The cocktail is best given early, within the first five to seven days—while the patient is in the flu stage. I have had success treating [patients], even as late as fourteen days, when [they] have been sent home, untreated from the ER.

The timing of the drug is when the virus is in the period of maximal replication in the upper respiratory tract. My goal is to prevent hospitalization, which was achieved by reevaluating high-risk patients every two to three days. I blend in corticosteroids and prolong the HCQ treatment for five to thirty more days if symptoms warrant, but they generally do not. I use it especially in high-risk individuals: those over sixty or with comorbidities and anyone with moderate to severe flu symptoms. The healthy do not need the treatment.

I used this regimen to successfully treat thirty-one elderly nursing home residents in an outbreak in June, and twenty-nine recovered fully. The drug works mechanistically through multiple actions: the ionophore HCQ (the "gun") and zinc ("the bullet"). HCQ blocks the sigma-1 receptor and has several other direct antiviral effects. The antibiotic also has an antiviral effect and potentiates the action of the HCQ and zinc. As additional anti-COVID agents become available, they can be added to this regimen to enhance its efficacy.

I am routinely now combining ivermectin in a quadruple HCQ/IVM cocktail with excellent results since ivermectin is safe and has a different anti-COVID action. Monoclonal antibodies from Regeneron and Lilly will be suitable also, when [they are] readily available.

The results are consistently good, often dramatic, with improvement within forty-eight hours. I have seen very few hospitalizations and only a few deaths in patients who were exceedingly sick to begin with—and received the medication late or while hospitalized.

I have not seen a single negative cardiac event and few other side effects, despite what we hear in the media. My experience is in line with all the studies regarding early use of the HCQ cocktail.

LET ME BE CLEAR: THIS IS ONLY ABOUT THE SCIENCE. THE SCIENCE OF VIRAL REPLICATION, THE SCIENCE OF THE STAGES OF COVID, AND THE SCIENCE of WHY EARLY TREATMENT WORKS.

The science tells us that early treatment would be an effective strategy to use on a national level, which motivated me and a few of my colleagues to write a letter to the President, a letter to my congressman, a letter to the California health department, an open letter to Dr. Fauci, and a national plan for COVID-19.

This is not about an opinion of an "expert." This is about science and data. As we describe in the National Plan, this approach would be the solution to the pandemic . . . [it would] protect the vulnerable, and if high-risk individuals get sick, there is a solution for them with early treatment with the antiviral cocktail.

If early treatment was available, people would be much more confident going back to work and sending their kids back to school.[14]

Although the Senate Homeland Security Committee convened the November 19th hearing, it was not televised nationally and was sparsely attended, even by its own committee members. Many in the medical and scientific community questioned why this was the

---

14   Fareed, G. (2020, November 25). "Statement of George Fareed, M.D. for Senate Hearing, November 19, 2020." *The Desert Review*. Retrieved November 17, 2021, from https://www.thedesertreview.com/news/statement-of-george-fareed-m-d-for-senate-hearing-november-19-2020/article_e80b17ce-2f3c-11eb-8cce-df403566aab9.html.

case. Surely, people would want to know if there was early, effective treatment for COVID-19. This disregard for information occurred right before the largest COVID spikes we saw in the country and the rest of the Northern Hemisphere.

The meeting provided essential insight into why the U.S. failed miserably in the medical management of COVID-19, especially with high-risk patients. Rather than embracing early treatment (which is how most illnesses are managed), the medical establishment, specifically academia and federal health agencies, has actively suppressed the evidence for early outpatient treatment of the COVID-19 illness. The two-and-a-half-hour hearing is essential viewing for all Americans, given that over 275,000, as of December 1, 2020, of our citizens have died and many aspects of society are being devastated by lockdowns. You can view the video here: https://www.c-span.org/video/?478159-1/ senate-hearing-covid-19-outpatient-treatment

Dr. McCullough, who directly treats COVID patients, described his scholarly article published in the *American Journal of Medicine* (August 2020) titled "Pathophysiological Basis and Rationale for Early Outpatient Treatment of SARS-CoV-2 (COVID-19) Infection."[15]

In his testimony, Dr. McCullough described the "four pillars of pandemic response," including "Contagion Control," "Early Home Treatment," "Hospitalization," and "Vaccination." He emphasized our collective medical response in sharp contrast to the media portrayal that has ignored early treatment.

McCullough then described the stages of COVID-19 illness to include viral replication, cytokine storm, and micro-thrombosis. He

---

15   Define_me (n.d.). Retrieved November 17, 2021, from https://www.amjmed.com/article/S0002-9343(20)30673-2/ fulltext.

discussed how early outpatient treatment is a multi-drug regimen to disrupt viral replication, thereby reducing the risk of progression to high-morbidity cytokine storm and micro-thrombosis.

Hydroxychloroquine (HCQ), the drug most familiar to the public, is one of several drugs in Dr. McCullough's published algorithm, not only to disrupt viral replication and packaging, but also to treat the ravaging effects of cytokine storm and micro-thrombosis.

Dr. Harvey Risch presented his analysis of the research involving early treatment, focusing on the outpatient use of hydroxychloroquine, because it is the most studied drug. Dr. Risch emphasized outpatient treatment of symptomatic high-risk patients within the first five to seven days of illness with the "HCQ cocktail," consisting of HCQ in combination with zinc and an antibiotic, azithromycin, or doxycycline. Dr. Risch has published a paper in the American Journal of Epidemiology analyzing the data.[16]

Risch's conclusion, drawn from established powerful and informative statistical methods (such as meta-analyses), is that early treatment of symptomatic, high-risk COVID-19 patients is both safe and dramatically effective.

While the hearing began with Sen. Johnson (the majority leader) providing background for the early treatment of symptomatic, high-risk COVID-19 patients, the minority leader for the hearing (Sen. Gary Peters; D-MI), did not mention early treatment once in his remarks.

Rather, Mr. Peters discussed legislation that would create a COVID-19 "disinformation and misinformation" task force, purportedly

16   HA;, R. (n.d.). "Early outpatient treatment of symptomatic, high-risk COVID-19 patients that should be ramped up immediately as key to the pandemic crisis." *American Journal of Epidemiology*. Retrieved November 17, 2021, from https://pubmed.ncbi.nlm.nih.gov/32458969/.

to control the spread of unfounded information and save American lives. He then said, in a veiled reference to the topic being discussed, "We must also be careful about giving Americans a false sense of security by promoting untested and unproven outpatient remedies."

Senator Peters and his colleagues did not pose one single question to the three physicians/scholars advocating for early outpatient treatment of symptomatic high-risk COVID-19 patients. All their questions were directed to Dr. Jha, "the minority expert," covering topics like testing capability, vaccination, and whether families should gather that year for Thanksgiving.

Dr. Ashish Jha, the dean of the School of Public Health at Brown University, rebutted during the forum as "the minority expert." Dr. Jha testified he has not treated COVID-19 patients. Dr. Jha, moreover, has no peer-reviewed articles on the treatment of COVID-19 illness.

To be clear, Dr. Jha was testifying as a purported "expert" in the early treatment of COVID-19 illness, yet he has no experience in treating COVID-19 patients and, unlike Drs. McCullough and Risch, has not produced a single peer-reviewed article on the subject.

Dr. Jha testified that his opinions were derived from his review of the scientific literature, stating none of the ostensibly "high-quality, randomized control trial studies" concluded that HCQ is effective in treating COVID-19 illness. He stated that observational studies were not of sufficient quality to conclude that HCQ is effective. He pointed out his opinions are in line with the consensus of experts in academia and are also in accordance with the opinions of the CDC, NIH, and FDA.

Unlike Dr. McCullough, Dr. Jha never discussed the science of COVID-19 illness in his remarks. In fact, he did not dispute Dr. McCullough's description of the different stages of the illness or the rationale for early treatment.

Oseltamivir/Tamiflu, by example, interferes with viral replication, disrupting the progression of influenza illness. Accordingly, as Dr. McCullough explained, if treatment can interfere with viral replication early in the course of COVID-19 illness, we can confidently prevent progression to higher morbidity stages of the disease.

Again, Dr. Jha did not challenge Dr. McCullough on the science, pathophysiologic, and pharmacologic basis of early treatment for all three facets of the disease: viral replication, cytokine storm, and thrombosis.

Dr. Jha and other recognized national "experts" such as Dr. Fauci do not offer any recommendations regarding early outpatient treatment of COVID-19 illness, which was the subject of the meeting in November 2020. Dr. Jha's intention was to deny the overwhelming evidence supporting early treatment with HCQ and ivermectin (IVM)-based protocols. Indeed, outpatient treatment extends far beyond the use of only HCQ. Dr. Jha did not address other aspects of Dr. McCullough's outpatient treatment protocol targeting the progression of COVID-19 illness to cytokine storm and micro-thrombosis.

There was an obvious flaw with Dr. Jha's argument against the use of HCQ and IVM: none of the randomized, control trials he cited involved early treatment within five to seven days of high-risk patients with the full HCQ or IVM cocktail. A cocktail, not just HCQ and/ or IVM alone, is used by doctors around the world to interfere with viral replication to prevent progression to cytokine storm and micro-thrombosis. Dr. Jha, however, never addressed the science of the virus and the well-described aspects of COVID-19 pathophysiology.

Moreover, he did not cite a single study disproving the approach of early treatment of high-risk patients. Dr. Jha's statement that "all the experts are in agreement" is not remotely sufficient in medical science polemics. Clinical conclusions and recommendations are based on rigorous data analysis and not merely consensus opinion.

In contrast, Dr. McCullough has over 600 peer-reviewed publications, including two dozen on COVID-19 disease. He has chaired many high-risk data safety monitoring boards and knows all the inner workings of large-scale clinical trials. Dr. Risch's expertise is in analyzing data from the literature and his renowned scholarship have resulted in over 300 peer-reviewed articles. As Dr. Risch emphasizes, all the studies involving early treatment of high-risk patients with HCQ have shown positive outcomes in reducing hospitalization and death.

In the recovery study cited by Dr. Jha, patients received HCQ when they were hospitalized with evolving or florid cytokine storm; the majority were on supplemental oxygen.[17]

The authors of another widely cited randomized control trial from Brazil on hospitalized patients (Cavalcanti et. al) concluded that if HCQ were given earlier, the results could have been different.[18]

The timing of pharmacological intervention is paramount when the goal is disruption of viral replication; it is all about the science, which Dr. Jha did not address in his testimony that day.

Dr. Jha also cited the Boulware et al. post-prophylaxis study from the University of Minnesota that was never brought to completion

---

[17] Fareed, G. (2020, November 25). "Statement of George Fareed, M.D. for Senate hearing, November 19, 2020." *The Desert Review*. Retrieved November 17, 2021, from https://www.thedesertreview.com/news/statement-of-george-fareed-m-d-for-senate-hearing-november-19-2020/article_e80b17ce-2f3c-11eb-8cce-df403566aab9.html.

[18] Cavalcanti, A. B., Al., E., for the Coalition Covid-19 Brazil I Investigators*, Author Affiliations From Hcor Research Institute (A.B.C., Others, N. E. L. C. and, Others, V. B. and, Others, N. C. and, E. B. Walter and Others, Monto, A. S., & F. P. Polack and Others. (2021, January 14). "Hydroxychloroquine with or without azithromycin in mild-to-moderate covid-19: Nejm." *New England Journal of Medicine*. Retrieved November 17, 2021, from https://www.nejm.org/doi/full/10.1056/NEJMoa2019014.

but published in the New England Journal of Medicine: a paper that showcases academic fraud regarding HCQ.[19]

The study looked at individuals who were exposed to COVID-19 and compared those receiving HCQ post-exposure with those who did not receive the medication. Although the study concluded that HCQ was not better than placebo in preventing an infection, the authors did not stratify the results as to when the HCQ was given; in fact, the raw data showed that those receiving HCQ earlier after exposure had a statistically significant decrease in infection (see analysis Watanabe, Brazil).[20]

These results were conveniently left out of the published study. Again, it is about the science and the critical timing of HCQ administration. The earlier a patient receives HCQ after an exposure, the better one's chances are to not develop a symptomatic infection. This is precisely what the study revealed, and yet the results supporting the conclusion were suspiciously omitted.

Dr. Jha's testimony that there is "overwhelming evidence" against the early, outpatient use of HCQ is false. He provided no evidence to support his opinion; in fact, no such evidence exists. The studies he cited (on hospitalized patients) do not disprove the early, outpatient use of HCQ, and what he presented is best described (using terminology from Sen. Peters) as "misinformation" and "disinformation."

In sharp contrast to Dr. McCullough's algorithm that focuses on a multi-drug regimen to address the different manifestations

---

19 Boulware, D. R., Al., E., Author AffiliationsFrom the University of Minnesota (D.R.B., Cohen, M. S., Others, N. E. L. C. and, Others, V. B. and, Others, N. C. and, E. B. Walter and Others, Monto, A. S., & F. P. Polack and Others. (2020, August 6). "A Randomized Trial of Hydroxychloroquine as Postexposure Prophylaxis for Covid-19." *New England Journal of Medicine*. Retrieved November 17, 2021, from https://www.nejm.org/doi/full/10.1056/NEJMoa2016638.

20 Watanabe, M. (2020, July 21). "Efficacy of Hydroxychloroquine as Prophylaxis for Covid-19." arXiv.org. Retrieved November 17, 2021, from https://arxiv.org/abs/2007.09477.

of COVID-19 infection, Dr. Jha ignored the science of the virus and focused on only one drug, HCQ. Dr. Jha did not offer a single recommendation for outpatient treatment—none! His testimony appeared to serve one purpose only: to discredit HCQ.

The most disconcerting aspect of Dr. Jha's testimony is the brazenly false assertion that HCQ is dangerous, even with moderate doses recommended for early outpatient treatment of high-risk patients with symptomatic COVID-19 illness. The Veterans' Administration study to which Dr. Jha referred involved hospitalized, sick patients who received high doses of HCQ.[21]

Dr. Jha did not acknowledge that HCQ has been used for sixty-five years for malaria and nearly as long for rheumatoid diseases, and yet he deemed it dangerous when used in moderate doses for short courses of typically one to two weeks, for early treatment of high-risk outpatients.

This false characterization by so-called "experts" such as Dr. Jha, who have not even treated a COVID-19 patient, has likely discouraged countless high-risk patients from seeking outcome-altering early treatment. Dr. McCullough is a cardiologist; unlike Dr. Jha, McCullough is highly experienced in drug safety evaluations from clinical trials and stated Dr. Jha's testimony is "reckless and dangerous."

It is alarming to consider how many Americans have already died and continue to die during this pandemic. We, along with Drs. McCullough and Risch, have dedicated ourselves to reducing fatal outcomes by advocating early outpatient treatment for high-risk COVID-19 patients.

---

21 Magagnoli J;Narendran S;Pereira F;Cummings T;Hardin JW;Sutton SS;Ambati J;. (n.d.). "Outcomes of hydroxychloroquine usage in United States veterans hospitalized with Covid-19." Retrieved from https://pubmed.ncbi.nlm.nih.gov/32511622/.

As Dr. McCullough stressed, many countries are using early outpatient treatment strategies with take-home treatment packets with HCQ and IVM-based regimens. There are websites (http://www.c19study.com/) that list publications from around the world regarding HCQ and COVID-19 illness, irrespective of the results/conclusions. Another website, HCQ Trial (http://www.hcqtrial.com/), compares the results in countries that use HCQ with those that do not. Yet another resource, Worldometer (https://www.worldometers.info/coronavirus/), features a particularly illustrative statistic, "deaths/million."

Everyone can see the facts for themselves that the statistics do not lie: America and many European countries have failed in their response to the pandemic.

The United States, along with most European countries, have some of the most troubling statistics in terms of "deaths/million," with deaths per million significantly higher than many less technologically-developed countries that rely on early treatment with HCQ.

According to HCQ Trial (http://www.hcqtrial.com/), countries using HCQ have death rates that are 70% lower, as compared to countries that do not use HCQ. These results align nicely with outcomes obtained by physicians such as Dr. Fareed, who (unlike Dr. Jha) actually treat COVID-19 patients.

Senator Peters, as stated in his opening statement, seeks to remove "misinformation" from the COVID-19 discussion. Ironically, "misinformation" is precisely what Dr. Jha is doing when he makes the unsubstantiated claim that HCQ is dangerous when used in moderate doses for early treatment of high-risk outpatients without a single study to support this conclusion.

"Misinformation" is visible in Dr. Jha's suggestion that there is no evidence to support the early use of HCQ, when the website C19

Study (http://www.c19study.com/) shows that 96% of studies on the early use of HCQ show positive results and outcomes. This is significant evidence! Certainly, Dr. Jha's testimony could be the first target for Sen. Peters' COVID-19 disinformation and misinformation legislation.

Dr. Risch concluded that the combined literature of observational and retrospective studies provides overwhelming evidence to support early treatment and that the benefit of early treatment of high-risk patients far outweighs the risk of medication side effects.

There is always a risk-benefit consideration when deciding to pursue a treatment. Television commercials for pharmaceuticals consume much of the airtime delineating potential side effects. The selection of pharmacologic/therapeutic interventions is a sacred and revered aspect of the physician-patient relationship. An informed patient should decide on treatment with their doctor. Dr. Jha's therapeutic nihilism does not give him the liberty to promulgate false information about HCQ-based treatment for COVID-19 illness.

The insistence on randomized clinical trials (RCTs) by Drs. Jha and Fauci, when the NIH abandoned RCTs with COVID-19 outpatients, is absurd during a pandemic in which Americans are dying at such a rapid rate. We are fighting a war, and the best interventions in such circumstances come from those who are engaged in the battle; thousands of providers like us, who are on the frontlines.

There was no clinical trial for using penicillin in World War II; waiting for such a study would have cost hundreds of thousands of lives. Some of the greatest advancements in trauma surgery were discovered literally on the battlefield, not by RCTs at prestigious academic institutions.

Senator Peters' proposed legislation to monitor and regulate COVID-19 misinformation would not apply to Dr. Jha, but rather to physicians with therapeutic recommendations that run counter to the desired narrative of self-proclaimed "experts."

Many of us have produced magnificent videos discussing the science of and rationale for early treatment of COVID-19 illness. But the videos were censored and labeled as "misinformation" by YouTube, Facebook, and Twitter, all without declaring what content of the presentations was allegedly not true. Senator Peters wants to address such blatant censorship in national policy. This is Orwellian!

The medical profession is best served when physicians challenge and question one another. Dr. Jha, meanwhile, resorts to CNN and MSNBC commentary with political pundits. Dr. Jha should discuss the science of proposed treatment protocols with categorical experts like Dr. McCullough, and frontline physicians with vast experience treating COVID-19 patients.

Dr. Jha neither considers the rationale for early treatment of COVID-19 illness nor discloses that many countries, including his native India, successfully manage the pandemic with HCQ, IVM, and favipiravir, combined with other drugs. If the naysayer "experts" are interested in saving lives, they would focus on early treatment, which is a hallmark and standard of care for physicians treating any identified disease or condition.

One should wonder why the committee minority could not find a single "expert" to testify under oath that HCQ or IVM-based treatment, when used early in the flu stage of COVID-19 illness, is ineffective and dangerous. In fact, such a physician-expert does not exist.

If there is truth to what Dr. Jha contends, countless physicians and patients would come forward with testimonial horror stories. CNN and MSNBC would gleefully invite such individuals to share their affirming experiences. Yet not a single case series in the published literature disputes that HCQ or IVM-based early treatment is safe and effective for high-risk COVID-19 patients.

This serves to reinforce the widespread use of HCQ and IVM-based early treatment for symptomatic COVID-19 illness in countries with scarce medical resources. The best Senator Peters could do was to bring an "expert" who speaks authoritatively but has never treated a COVID-19 patient and has the chutzpah on social media and with the mainstream media to castigate physicians, who risk their lives treating COVID-19 patients, for spreading "misinformation" and "not following the science."

This is a clarion call for America to wake up! To have arrived at this point of suffering and death while rejecting evidence-based early, life-saving treatment options is simply bone-chilling.

The aftermath of the hearing is telltale. Dr. Jha appeared on multiple cable network shows and gave interviews to multiple publications with the same sinister narrative which was that Drs. McCullough, Fareed, and Risch are spreading misinformation. Dr. Jha's opinion piece in the New York Times is a must-read and is thoroughly revealing.

In this piece, Dr. Jha never discusses the science of the virus or conclusive evidence of the reduction in disease progression or hospitalizations with early treatment. Dr. Jha does not discuss any drug except hydroxychloroquine, ignoring the pathophysiology and pharmacologic principles heralded by Dr. McCullough, upon which a safe and effective early treatment multidrug regimen is based.

The most egregious and unconscionable accusation by Dr. Jha, however, is that those of us who testified, as well as Senator Johnson, are "snake oil salesmen."[22] Dr. Jha, who has never treated a single

---

22 Jha, A. (2020, November 24). "The Snake-Oil Salesmen of the Senate." *The New York Times*. Retrieved November 17, 2021, from https://www.nytimes.com/2020/11/24/opinion/hydroxychloroquine-covid.html.

COVID-19 patient, is compelled to denigrate physician-scholars who risk their lives and give hope by treating acutely ill COVID-19 patients.

As if the fifty-dollar drug cocktail is making these physicians money! With far too many Americans dead, one would hope that physicians like Dr. Jha would be supportive of physicians "in the field" who offer safe and effective early treatment for COVID-19 illness. Shame on Dr. Jha and Brown University!

Why would Dr. Jha so vehemently oppose a safe, inexpensive, effective, readily-available treatment that doctors around the world are using with demonstrable success, and at the same time offer no alternative other than to wait for a vaccine? With evidence-based safety and efficacy, why not allow a symptomatic, high-risk COVID-19 patient to decide with their physician how they want to be treated, as in all areas of medicine?

To find an answer, one needs to "follow the money." Dr. Jha, as documented in his appointment announcement at Brown University, receives funding from the Bill and Melinda Gates Foundation, which is championing a vaccine.[23]

Early treatment would be perceived by many Americans as an alternative to a vaccine. Dr. Jha has a clear conflict of interest that he did not disclose in his sworn Senate testimony, New York Times op-ed piece, and during numerous television appearances.

Unlike Dr. Jha, there is no conflict of interest for physicians who use inexpensive, generic medications and nutraceuticals to save the lives of patients with COVID-19 illness. Senator Peters and his colleagues squandered a glaring opportunity to expose alleged "disinformation and misinformation" from the assembled physician/scholars who

---

23 The Office of the Provost. (n.d.). Retrieved from https://www.brown.edu/about/administration/provost/communications/announcement-school-public-health-dean.

were recommending early outpatient treatment. If the physician/ scholars were promoting "untested and unproven" treatments, as Peters suggested, this was the opportunity to question them in front of the American people—but they did not.

In Pravda-like fashion, the mainstream media, such as the New York Times, CNN, and MSNBC, are complicit in advancing Dr. Jha's patently false narrative to the public without a contrasting evidence-based discussion from those who actually treat COVID-19 patients and are following the science.

UNSTOPPABLE

As the months passed, we knew we needed to keep our message alive and relevant. In addition to our impassioned pleas to Congress, we took another step forward by participating in the Reopen California Now public policy convention. Here is a recap of that powerful event, which was published in the *Calexico Chronicle*:

> *Over the weekend of January 8, 2021, Fareed was one of several healthcare experts taking part in the Reopen California Now public policy convention in the gated Sacramento neighborhood of Rancho Murieta.*
>
> *Speakers from the medical field were joined by state law enforcement officials and economic experts arguing that the California economy should be reopened immediately, despite record numbers of COVID-19 deaths and hospitalizations.*
>
> *The event ran from Friday, Jan. 8, through Sunday, Jan. 10, with the bulk of the discussion occurring during sessions on Saturday, when Fareed was part of a panel discussion.*

Many of the views shared at the conference are considered controversial and outside the mainstream. The event was webcast over Reopen California Now's Facebook page. Despite all the data presented and experts on site, the State of California chose not to reinstate in-person learning in schools; they did not open up the state until June 15, 2021, and state officials re-implemented mask policies even for the vaccinated populace in August.

Fareed, who has gained national exposure during the pandemic for his advocacy on early COVID interventions, such as the widespread use of a hydroxychloroquine cocktail, was included in a Q&A session focusing on the science behind COVID-19 and possible treatments for the virus.

He spoke alongside University of California, Los Angeles' Dr. Joe Ladapo, and entrepreneur Steve Kirsch. Dr. Jay Bhattacharya was also one of the guest speakers. Dr. Bhattacharya is one of the authors of the Great Barrington Declaration, a statement drafted by the American Institute for Economic Research, a free-market think tank in Great Barrington, Massachusetts.

Their statement calls for the reopening of the national economy and for those who are not at a significant risk of dying from COVID-19 to resume their normal daily lives and for those who are at risk to be intensely shielded from the virus. The statement posits that a high transmission rate among lower-risk individuals would lead to "herd immunity" for those at higher risk.

The World Health Organization, along with dozens of other national health organizations, has refuted the claims made in that statement and claim the herd immunity component alone would be undermined by the limited post-infection immunity period and it would be impossible to shield all of those who are vulnerable from contracting the virus. In a published interview, infectious disease specialist Anthony Fauci called the Barrington Declaration "nonsense and very dangerous."

Fareed and Bhattacharya both called for the early treatment of COVID-19 using cocktails of drugs that have not yet been widely accepted by the larger medical community as effective against the virus, including HCQ and the antidepressant fluvoxamine, which has antiviral action for COVID-19. They also spoke of humanized monoclonal antibodies, two therapies of which were recently awarded U.S. Food and Drug Administration emergency-use authorization.

"The monoclonal antibodies are excellent therapeutics, and if they could be given early and with convalescent plasma (another antibody treatment), if it's given in the early window, within the first three days of the onset of symptoms, there is a definite benefit," Fareed said, adding that he believes the use of the experimental treatment should be more widespread in urgent-care centers and clinical settings.

"They are expensive," Fareed acknowledged. "However, the U.S. government (U.S. taxpayers) has paid for them so individuals for now don't incur their costs."

For now, the FDA-authorized monoclonal antibody treatments are only being administered through hospitals, but to outpatients within ten days of COVID diagnosis.

With early-intervention medications and experimental treatments, Fareed claimed there have been efforts to suppress knowledge and distribution of these therapies during the COVID crisis.

"For me, the worst thing has been this suppression of early treatment and the consideration of a number of agents that can

suppress the early viral replication and allow the at-risk individuals not to be hospitalized and die," he said. "As they become available, they should be tested thoroughly and combined and used, and they should have been offered from the get-go and should not have been stigmatized."

Fareed said he has received some backlash for suggesting these drugs should be used, but that he has "ignored totally any reaction against me." He said he had been "picked upon" by Imperial County Health Department officials for using HCQ to treat nursing-home patients during an outbreak at Imperial Heights Healthcare and Wellness Centre in Brawley during the summer. He added that had he known about it, he also would have used fluvoxamine as part of the treatments.

"I've felt (backlash) from people in the community, or doctors even who have not wanted to do anything, that have accepted this 'don't do anything' approach, and 'you're going to do more harm if anything,' and I've just ignored it," Fareed said.

"And I'm isolated in a rural area on my own, and I've seen the truth. I've seen the patients improve and the expressions, and maybe agents like fluvoxamine are going to be even faster in achieving that. Whatever it is, I will use it," he added.

Bhattacharya called for open communication on the subject and said that he regrets the way that Fareed has been treated.

"I really regret that you've been attacked in the way that you have," he said. "It is a failure of our professional responsibility if we don't say what we see. What I've learned from the Great Barrington Declaration is that there are a lot of people that think like we do, they're just cowed into silence because they don't want to face the press attacking you, misrepresenting you, accusing you of things you

don't believe, which has all happened to me. But there's no other choice—we have to speak up. Millions of lives are at stake here."[24]

It is important to note that Dr. Tyson also brought up the EUA policy and the condition of use: "Under that policy, in order to get a medication or product an EUA there must 'be no adequate, approved or alternative to the candidate product for diagnosing, preventing or treating the disease or condition.'[25] This was revealing in that was this the reason they did not want repurposed drugs that are cheap, to be taken off the market for this disease ONLY?"

Dr. Tyson continued: "Knowing that the experimental drug remdesivir was coming, convalescent plasma, monoclonal antibodies, and the experimental vaccine. They all came in under the EUA policy. Had hydroxychloroquine and ivermectin been approved for use, that would eliminate the ability to use any of those treatments and thus eliminate the billions of dollars made off the experimental treatments listed above."

24 News, I. C., Luke Phillipson January 13, 2., Also, S., News, I. R., Marcie Landeroson October 26, 2., Katherine Ramoson November 21, 2., . . . Julio Morales and Richard Montenegro BrownPublic SafetyRegional News. (2021, January 13). "Dr. Fareed Talks Early Treatment at Re-Open Cal Now." Retrieved from https://calexicochronicle.com/2021/01/13/dr-fareed-talks-early-treatment-at-re-open-cal-now/.

25 "Emergency Use Authorization of Medical Products." (n.d.). Retrieved from https://www.fda.gov/media/97321/download.

YOU DECIDE

Taking all of this information into account, we urge every American to watch the Senate Homeland Security Committee hearing of 19 November 2020 (https://www.c-span.org/video/?478159-1/senate-hearing-covid-19-outpatient-treatment) and draw your own conclusions. Note which physician-scholars are focused on the medicine and the science of COVID-19, and who avoids discussing the science. See who is offering an evidence-based outpatient treatment for symptomatic high-risk COVID-19 patients, and who is not proposing any solution, except to go home and "wait and see."

See which politicians are for censorship and who is for an open discussion, and which politicians refuse to discuss early treatment for symptomatic COVID-19 patients. We believe that you will have an informed perspective as to why there are around 275,000 dead Americans when other countries with considerably fewer resources have fared much better.

CHAPTER 6

WHY THE VACCINE APPROACH HAS FAILED AND WILL LIKELY CAUSE MORE HARM THAN GOOD

While rejecting early treatment, the leaders of the pandemic response have embraced a two-pronged approach: (1) attempting to avoid infections through social distancing/masking and mass vaccination, and (2) mass vaccination. Aside from the fact that lockdowns and social distancing were devastating in so many ways, the rationale for this approach was to minimize the number of infections until a vaccine came along that could wipe out the virus. That was the plan.

Unless one is in denial, by all objective measures this plan has failed. Even with a vaccination program that has resulted in over 65% of adults "fully vaccinated" and even a higher percentage in those over seventy years of age, there have been more deaths in 2021 than in 2020 when there was no vaccine. People are told to continue to socially distance and wear masks as the public health officials panic the public about the next variant. More lockdowns are threatened. Life is anything but normal.

This is a very different picture than what was promised. In fact, the United States and all the other Western countries that have rejected early treatment and relied on vaccines have failed in their response to COVID-19 as compared to countries with far fewer resources. One study showed that the 65 countries and the 2,400 counties in the United State with the highest vaccination rates had the highest number of cases. All one has to do is to go to "Worldometer.com" and look at the charts on coronavirus—the least advanced countries have done much better in terms of "deaths/million." How could this have happened?

In one word, "science."

It all starts with the knowledge that the original experimental trial with the Pfizer vaccine (as well as Moderna) showed approximately a 95% effectiveness in reducing infections . . . that's 95% and not 100%. While this may have seemed promising, this should have been a "red flag" for those under the belief that mass vaccination would end the pandemic. This is because a vaccine that is 95% effective in preventing an infection is an "imperfect" or "leaky" vaccine. We have accumulated knowledge about "leaky vaccines," and should have known that such an approach would not end the pandemic.

An article in the Journal of Science in 2001 discusses the phenomenon of an "imperfect vaccine."[26] The article states that "vaccines

---

26   Gandon, S., Mackinnon, M. J., Nee, S. & Read, A. F. "Imperfect vaccines and the evolution of pathogen virulence." *Nature* (2001). 414, 751-756.

designed to reduce pathogen growth rate and/or toxicity diminish selection of virulent pathogens. The subsequent evolution leads to higher levels of intrinsic virulence and hence more severe disease in unvaccinated individuals. *This evolution can erode population-wide benefits such that overall mortality rates are unaffected, or even increase, with the level of vaccination coverage.*[26] In contrast, infection-blocking vaccines induce no such effects, and can even select for lower virulence. The findings have policy implications, for the use and development of vaccines that are not expected to provide full immunity, such as candidates for malaria."

So, a "leaky vaccine" not only does not eliminate the spread of a viral infection, but it also generates variants that can be more lethal, especially to the unvaccinated. This concept was illustrated in a 2015 experiment in chickens with Marek's disease.[27] The data showed that "anti-disease vaccines that do not prevent transmission can create conditions that promote the emergence of pathogen strains that cause more disease in unvaccinated hosts."

The concept of what has occurred with COVID-19 is very basic: a virus will mutate to evade the antibodies created from a vaccine. We all know this concept from antibiotics. The more antibiotics are used, the more there are antibiotic-resistant strains created that are more dangerous (e.g., methicillin-resistant staphylococcus aureus "MRSA"). While antibiotics are a great tool in fighting bacterial infections, if used too much, they become much less effective.

The response to this vaccine strategy failure? Well, of course, more vaccinations in the form of "boosters." Now that we are hearing of a new variant, "Omicron", the knee-jerk response is—you guessed it, the

27   Read et. al. 2015 Biology Plos

need for more boosters. Dr. Fauci estimates that 70% of Americans will need to get the booster to prevent the spread of Omicron . . . and yet, there is no evidence as of yet that this variant is even dangerous. It is not just about more boosters. Once again, the approach is lockdowns and travel restrictions, as well as adding in the absolutely non-sensical measure of separating vaccinated from unvaccinated (e.g., Germany).

This failed approach brings to mind the famous quote by Dr. Albert Einstein, "The definition of insanity is doing the same thing over and over and expecting different results."

It takes quite a bit of brainwashing of a population to obtain compliance to a strategy that is so unscientific and insane. This requires ignoring the science, such as denying the effectiveness of natural immunity. There are now over 125 studies showing that natural immunity is at least as good or probably better than the vaccine (Brownstone institute.) This includes studies out of such places as the Cleveland Clinic, Emory, and Washington University.

An Israeli study showed that natural immunity is at least thirteen times more powerful than vaccination at preventing infection.[28] The CDC countered with a study of its own looking at hospitalized patients that concluded that vaccination was five times more powerful than natural immunity. This study was admittedly highly flawed: there was a full page in the discussion section of the "limitations" of the study. Dr. Martin Kuhldorf, an epidemiologist from Harvard, offered an analysis of the two studies that is a must-read for anyone who doubts the deception of the CDC.

---

28 Gazit, Sivan M.D. M.A., et al. "Comparing SARS-CoV-2 natural immunity to vaccine-induced immunity: reinfections versus breakthrough infections." Medrxiv. 2021.

Obviously, our public agencies cannot admit that their strategy has failed, so they need a scapegoat, a group to blame for prolonging the pandemic. We all know this to be "the Unvaccinated." The mass media propaganda campaign has now called this "the Pandemic of the Unvaccinated." This characterization, is, of course, false.

While the unvaccinated are at increased risk of severe illness and death (as seen in the Marek chicken study), the scientific evidence shows that the peak viral loads are very similar but the duration of viremia or virus shedding appears shortened in the vaccinated. Reports out of Israel and the UK showed a large fraction of new COVID-19 cases were occurring in vaccinated individuals. This fact explains why no country has been able to eradicate the virus through vaccination, as seen in countries such as Ireland and Denmark with vaccination rates approaching 90%.

So, mass vaccination does not stop the spread of COVID-19. Moreover, it comes with a cost that is ignored by our public health officials. In fact, bringing this subject up gets one labeled as a "conspiracy theorist." That subject is—adverse reactions caused by the vaccines.

This sets a vicious cycle in motion: countries that did not embrace early treatment will need to impose new waves of lockdowns. COVID-19 will begin surging again as it has been, and entire populations will once again be overwhelmed. This is what happened with Delta and other variants, as officials failed to treat early and instead merely continued to hope for miracles with genetic spike protein vaccines.

The deadly decisions agencies made early on have come back to haunt us. They stigmatized HCQ and recommended no early treatment protocols, while ignoring hundreds of efficacy studies—and COVID-19 has still been pervasive worldwide. New information and comparison studies have shown natural immunity is many times greater than vaccinated immunity against the Delta variant (and in all likelihood any new variants). This information should be regarded as good news as we approach a new herd immunity. In fact, studies on children 18 and under showed very few if any healthy children died from COVID-19 in 2020-2021.[29,30] These results support not vaccinating those age groups, as adverse effects would certainly not be worth the risk.

Unfortunately, the masses have been encouraged to vaccinate children, despite the overwhelming adverse effects that have been reported. These adverse effects include death. The government's VAERS (Vaccine Adverse Event Reporting System) is maintained by the CDC, and it is punishable with fines for uploading false information. The VAER has reported upwards of 18,000 deaths and over half a million adverse reactions from COVID vaccines. These numbers have never been seen before in the history of vaccines. This vaccine is responsible for more deaths than all vaccines combined over the last ten years.

But the vaccine is not just dangerous for children. What most people do not realize is that the spike protein is what is pathogenic (toxic) by itself, and it confers this toxicity when it is a part of the intact COVID-19 virus. In fact, the spike protein is exactly what makes the vaccine so disturbing. Knowing how pathogenic this protein is, why would doctors and scientists manufacture a vaccine that produces the spike protein in our own cells—and risk circulating that toxin in our bodies?

The human immune system can attack and kill those cells, no matter where they are. However, if those cells enter the vascular

---

29 Deaths by Sex, Ages 0-18 years. (n.d.). Retrieved from https://data.cdc.gov/NCHS/Deaths-by-Sex-Ages-0-18-years/xa4b-4pzv.

30 Foundation, T. H. (n.d.). COVID-19 Deaths by Age. Retrieved from https://datavisualizations.heritage.org/public-health/covid-19-deaths-by-age/.

system, the body's response can cause blood clots. When those cells enter the heart, myocarditis, and pericarditis can result, as the body tries to ward off those toxic cells.

In the nervous system and brain, the spike protein can cause strokes, Guillain-Barré Syndrome, Bell's palsy, neuropathies, and even transverse myelitis. Why would anyone choose an experimental vaccine with those possible side effects, even if those side effects are relatively rare?

FROM DR. FAREED: TRUE STORIES

Consider just a few of the victims' tragic stories, after they listened to the government and received a vaccine:

One of our patients was given the Pfizer vaccine in March 2021. After her first shot, she had suffered no major side effects, except for some flu-like symptoms. However, the day after her second shot, she passed away. The official cause of death was documented as a heart attack, but the spike protein from the vaccine can actually spread from the injection site to trigger clotting and vascular abnormalities in other organs. In this case, the family reported this tragedy to VAERS—yet that won't bring their beloved mother and mother-in-law back: someone who could have lived many more healthy, happy years if she had not succumbed to the adverse side effects of the vaccine.[31]

Another patient already had COVID and had been successfully treated with the HCQ protocol; however, she still decided to get vaccinated (despite the fact that her body had already created natural antibodies). After her first dose, she was extremely sick, with a fever, vomiting, and simply feeling ill in general. She had a similar reaction after the second dose—and mentioned how it felt like she had gotten COVID all over again.[32]

31   https://twitter.com/GeorgeFareed2/status/14110129656087879970?s=20
32   https://twitter.com/GeorgeFareed2/status/14110149884587721281?s=20

A nurse who received her second Moderna jab experienced sickness for a week. Even after the other side effects subsided, her asthmatic symptoms were exacerbated—not just for a week, but for months! Despite taking steroids and other medications to alleviate her symptoms, she can't get over these asthma indications.[33]

Yet another woman spoke to us about her coworker, who had a solitary kidney. This woman's single kidney, which previously functioned at 65%, fell to 9% within the first week after her vaccination. Fortunately, she is feeling better now—but at what cost are we willing to allow people to get pressured into getting the vaccine, knowing the adverse side effects this can cause in certain individuals?[34]

A THOUGHTFUL RESPONSE

On November 2, 2021, Senator Ron Johnson held a panel discussion with doctors and medical researchers who have treated COVID-19 patients' vaccine injuries. These heroes are researching the safety and efficacy of the COVID-19 vaccines, and they shared what they are learning during this discussion. The panel also included patients who experienced adverse events following vaccination, and family members who lost loved ones needlessly to a vaccine that is dangerous and toxic.

Yes, the vaccine propaganda machine and subsequent mandates are putting incredible pressure on citizens to "do their part" to "stop the spread." Sadly, the government, medical establishment, and academia have not been transparent in the potentially lethal side effects that this new vaccine can cause. Watch the video (https://www.youtube.com/watch?v=lkVN3KwDfvI) and—as with the Congressional testimony—draw your own conclusions.

33   https://twitter.com/GeorgeFareed2/status/1413712939085819904?s=20
34   https://twitter.com/GeorgeFareed2/status/1400229914587009028?s=20

Vaccine injury is real. Vaccine deaths are a horrific "side effect" that nobody wants to talk about. This is why, during that panel discussion, Senator Johnson asked this important question we all should ponder: "How can you help them [citizens] recover, if you're not willing to admit vaccine injuries are real?"

FROM DR. TYSON: THERE ARE TOO MANY QUESTIONS . . . BUT THERE'S A BETTER WAY

There are still way too many questions about this vaccine for anyone to feel comfortable mandating that everyone receives the vaccine. I explain in detail why I feel so strongly about this topic in the following *The Desert Review article:*

Dr. Brian Tyson, a parent and medical doctor who founded the All Valley Urgent Care with offices in El Centro and Brawley, spoke on several issues and background information surrounding COVID-19.

Even before the family physician had reached the podium, some in the audience called out to yield their 3-minute time allotment to Dr. Tyson. Their gestures meant additional time for the doctor to speak more than his allotted time.

Dr. Tyson introduced himself as a COVID-19 expert recognized across the nation and at the international level. He came back from Washington D.C. the previous day, after meeting with Senator Rand Paul (Kentucky), Senator Ron Johnson (Wisconsin), and Congressman Mark Meadows (North Carolina).

"OSHA announced that a circuit court order will suspend implementation and enforcement of the vaccination mandate," said Dr. Tyson, referring to the Occupational Safety and Health Administration.

Dr. Tyson informed board members, "There is still no FDA approved vaccine available in the USA."

And on the subject of voluntary consent, Dr. Tyson referred to the Nuremberg Code which he read from his cell phone: "It made voluntary consent a requirement in clinical research studies—emphasizing that consent can be voluntary only if participants are able to consent, they are free from coercion, for example—outside pressure, and must comprehend the risks and benefits involved."

Dr. Tyson asked, "Has anybody seen the vaccine insert? It says, 'Intentionally left blank.' It means that nobody knows what the risks and benefits are. There is no informed consent. So, then, the vaccine should be a decision between the patient and the provider, not a state mandate."

"Anyone should be afforded that personal choice based on their risk factors, based on their co-morbidities, based on their decision to take medical treatment or not, under the emergency use authorization statute upheld by the FDA."

"Mandates need to go away. This is a free society," said Dr. Tyson. He also offered his help and any assistance needed to board members regarding the issue."[35]

Like Senator Johnson, I believe that the time for transparency is well overdue. There's a better way to handle this pandemic, and at the global COVID summit in San Juan, Puerto Rico September 6-8, 2021, I shared some of my views:

It's not a diagnosis of COVID. It's a diagnosis of inflammation, pneumonia . . . nausea . . . and diarrhea; getting people monoclonal antibodies . . . early on . . . has been shown to have a huge improvement. I've seen, from 2 months to 102 years old . . . I've seen unvaccinated . . . to vaccinated . . . to even booster vaccinated positive patients—but the one thing is, they all respond to treatment. And I think that's the biggest lesson that everybody needs to hear. Early treatment is so crucial and they need to stop blocking us from saving people's lives.

35   Villero, J. N. (2021, November 22). "More letters to Newsom opposing COVID mandates." Retrieved from https://www.thedesertreview.com/health/more-letters-to-newsom-opposing-covid-mandates/article_16125000-4b71-11ec-99f5-db2208129daf.html.

My colleague, Dr. Fareed, wholeheartedly agrees, and at the International COVID Summit in Rome, Italy, he shared those views.

FROM DR. FAREED: THE ROME SUMMIT

Dr. Robert Malone, inventor of the mRNA platform technology, convened the International COVID Summit in Rome, Italy. I was fortunate to be among one of the elite invited speakers. Below are excerpts from my introductory and closing remarks to the Italian Senate on September 13, 2021:

Dear Senators, colleagues, friends, ladies, and gentlemen, it's a great honor for me to address you today. I graduated in 1970 from Harvard University Medical School. Yes, my medical career now exceeds fifty years, and it encompasses a variety of aspects of medicine, including research in virology and immunology, but most importantly, family medicine.

Today, I am a proud family physician. I believe in family medicine. Everyone should have a qualified, caring family physician who will focus on prevention and early treatment of any disease. And COVID should never have been different. It's a disease that can be prevented and treated early.

No one needs to die from COVID.

Ladies and gentlemen, I am humbled to be here. This may be the most important speech of my life.

Yes, I could speak about all the wrongs of the response of our respective governments to the pandemic. I could talk for hours and hours about these egregious mistakes. But despite all these wrongs, despite the tragedy that is still unfolding, despite the numerous hurdles we encounter for practicing good medicine, I want this to be a message of hope.

I want us to continue to fight the good fight. We must fight together for good medicine; we must fight together for the lifesaving protocols used in prevention and early treatment of COVID.

One and a half years ago, in March 2020, I began administering early treatments for patients with COVID. Along with my colleague Brian Tyson, we have now treated well over 7,000 patients.

From my experience, let me state it boldly: no one needs to die from COVID. No one should die from COVID. COVID is a treatable disease. If we treat COVID early, no one dies.

Let me repeat: If we treat COVID early, no one dies.

Yes, unfortunately, we experienced a few deaths in our practice. But it was with patients who presented at our clinics too late, or who did not adhere to the treatment protocol, or preferred to seek hospital care, where we have no influence on treatment.

All the patients we treated early, and who adhered to our treatments, lived. They were mostly adults with comorbidities. Sometimes, we treated elderly people, in their eighties or nineties. We treated only a few children, as they rarely develop a severe disease.

The vast majority of our patients presented early and adhered to our treatment. It's extremely fulfilling for me as a physician fulfilling my Hippocratic Oath, to tell you they all survived COVID, as they presented early and received treatment.

This is what I observed from the very beginning in March 2020. Yes, the disease has evolved with the variants, but our understanding of the disease, and the early, pre-hospital treatment protocols have also improved considerably.

It's why I can firmly state that no one needs to die from COVID. This should be our message. And we need to proclaim it, clearly and emphatically, to the world.

In early 2020, while the epidemic was already raging here in Italy, we had just a few cases in California, so we had a bit of time to prepare.

We quickly learned and adapted from the work and studies of Professor Didier Raoult in France and Dr. Vladimir Zelenko in New York: two doctors I admire and who brought us, already in March 2020, what became the basis of an effective treatment for COVID.

In developing our treatment protocols, I had long discussions with my amazing colleague, Dr. Brian Tyson. We also consulted with the AAPS, the American Association of Physicians and Surgeons, and its leader, the amazing Dr. Peter McCullough, concerning the early treatment of COVID.

When COVID did strike in Southern California, we were ready, and we were able to confidently begin using a calculated treatment protocol. This treatment protocol, which evolved with time, has retrospectively proven to be effective—extraordinarily effective.

Partnerships with the general population, as well as with our patients, proved to be extremely important. In the beginning, there was skepticism in the community. But quickly, word of the successes of early treatment spread. The narrative became: "If you have COVID symptoms, and you get treatment with Dr. Tyson or Dr. Fareed, they will take care of you— and the chances are high you will not be admitted to the hospital."

The residents of our rural, predominantly low-income area quickly understood hospital treatment often led to a one-way street to death—and was to be avoided at all costs. They were right. Hospital mortality rates were high, and even now, in many hospitals, it remains high. Too high. Even if some hospitals have adopted much-improved treatment protocols.

In the interest of educating our fellow citizens, Dr. Tyson also taught training sessions about COVID prevention in corporations. Corporations don't want their employees sick or absent. Due to this training, we believe many businesses played an important role in sending us patients who were suffering from their initial COVID symptoms.

But Dr. Tyson's urgent care clinic is not a large operation. Due to the high volume and rapid spread of the virus, we quickly and literally invaded the parking lot in front of his clinic and installed a triage tent. Many people lined up for diagnosis and treatment while waiting in their cars. Soon, we were more efficient than a McDonald's drive-through as we diagnosed our patients and prescribed them the appropriate treatment!

Often, we saw 300 or more patients in a single day, all with a limited staff of two doctors, four nurse practitioners, five nurses, four lab and x-ray technicians, and office support staff. It was epic. And proved, a small operation can diagnose and treat considerable numbers of patients. We did follow-ups with our patients by phone. And in some cases, we also worked through telemedicine.

In the U.S., Canada, France, and many countries, a significant amount of COVID outbreaks, severe disease, and death occurred in nursing homes. As the medical director for the Imperial Heights nursing home in Brawley, CA, I witnessed a major outbreak of *thirty-one patients presenting with and suffering COVID symptoms at the height of the pandemic in June 2020.*

With this outbreak raging, I intervened with our protocol, with the consent of the patients and/or their families. Most residents survived, although unfortunately, two died. Perhaps I should have intervened earlier, but it was difficult, due to the negative publicity about hydroxychloroquine at the time.

At the request of Jean-Pierre Kiekens from Covexit.com, who actually helped me prepare this speech, I have since written a protocol for the prevention and early treatment of COVID in nursing homes, relying on hydroxychloroquine (HCQ), ivermectin (IVM), and other agents.

For nursing homes, prevention is key and remains important even with vaccination, as there are so many breakthrough cases.

Presently, our regular treatment protocol comprises HCQ, IVM, doxycycline, zinc, vitamin D3, aspirin, and monoclonal antibodies. We follow the treatment algorithm developed by Professor Peter McCullough and his American and Italian colleagues.

We know this is the way to treat COVID. There is no doubt about it. We know it's the way to avoid severe disease and its repercussions. We know it's the way to avoid hospital admissions. We know it's the way to avoid long-term COVID and extended recoveries. We know.

Our results: we saved 99.96 percent of 4,576 symptomatic patients we treated, according to the draft of a retrospective study conducted by Mathew Crawford about our work.

We know early treatment works. We know early treatment is safe.

It is a disgrace this is not the standard of care for COVID in the U.S. and globally.

It is more than a disgrace. It's a tragedy.

With my fifty years of experience in medicine, I know, of course, about vaccines. I support safe and effective vaccines. And I personally have administered hundreds of thousands of them.

Regarding COVID, I have known since the beginning vaccines were not really necessary [and they] would be difficult to develop. [In addition, knowing that] there was absolutely no good reason to suppress early treatment in order to open the way for mass vaccination, I was optimistic the vaccines would help us tackle this pandemic.

I was vaccinated early on. I had not previously had COVID. And it was a group decision within the medical team of the hospital where I work, in addition to my collaboration with Dr. Tyson at his urgent care, and also the nursing home.

However, my perspective today on COVID vaccination has changed. I personally witnessed too many vaccine injuries—some fatal. I have seen the VAERS voluntary reporting data. I have read estimates on the actual numbers of adverse events. The data are clear: these are the most unsafe vaccines in the history of medicine.

We are living a new tragedy as we administer unsafe vaccines to healthy people, including children, who would most likely never develop severe disease or die from COVID if they receive early treatment. Far too many times, there are adverse events, serious adverse events, sometimes death, from these injections, and this is a tragedy.

In addition, I actually see fully vaccinated people in hospitals, because they had the false impression they were fully protected from COVID, when they were not. The authorities have called these cases "breakthrough" cases. They are actually cases of vaccine failure. And they are not rare. This is a new tragedy that was, again, avoidable if the authorities had done the right thing. In February 2021, there were clear signals these vaccines were not safe, but the campaign continues, despite the horrible safety signals stemming from reporting systems in the U.S., Europe, and the UK.

Today, the science is very clear. People [are] developing COVID-secure natural immunity. They develop robust, durable, natural immunity against COVID. This is better and more effective than the vaccine, because it is not limited to the spike protein.

So, in a sense, someone treated early for COVID, even with mild symptoms of the disease, will receive great natural immunities. In a sense, early treatment is a vaccine for COVID, and is much safer than the current vaccines.

I hope, one day, truly safe and effective vaccines against COVID will be developed. But today, such vaccines do not exist, and I am extremely concerned by the continued denial of this very fact by the authorities and their continued, unquestioned, mass vaccination policies, the various mandates, vaccination passes, and other measures implemented to essentially force vaccination on everyone.

I believe vaccines are intertwined with U.S. politics, and this is reprehensible. The former president, Donald Trump, pushed for the rapid development of the vaccines, in the belief he was doing the right thing: it would save lives.

Our current President, Joe Biden, continues the same policy and is pushing for mass vaccination, including youth, who are at nearly zero risk from the disease, as well as advocating for booster shots, because of the waning effectiveness of vaccines.

This political push for mass vaccination has caused official agencies in the U.S. and elsewhere to cease acknowledgment of the considerable and real safety issues.

In addition, there is considerable disinformation being promoted about early treatment, causing most medical doctors to not prescribe them; many now believe viable early treatments do not even exist. In actuality, they are by far the best way to handle this disease.

Medicine is in a very sad place today. Never in the history of medicine has it been advised that the best course is to not treat a disease in its early stages. Never has it been stated, in modern medicine, that someone should not be treated early and instead be left alone at home, fighting a deadly disease, without any form of treatment. Never. This is unconscionable.

Today, there is massive disinformation being disseminated among the population. Our patients are told the vaccines are safe and effective, and they are being indoctrinated that there is no early home treatment for COVID. Nothing could be further from the truth.

What we are told contradicts the facts. The truth is, early treatment works exceptionally well, and vaccines, in their current versions, are NOT safe and are much less effective in preventing severe disease and death than the early treatments. That is the truth.

My friends. I am just a seventy-seven-year-old family doctor. Never would I think I would one day come to such prominence, testifying before the U.S. Senate, commenting on national television in front of millions of viewers, or addressing [you] here in Rome during this prominent International COVID Summit.

I may be only a seventy-seven-year-old family doctor, but I am determined, I am strong, and I encourage you all to be determined and strong. We must be.

This goes beyond medicine. It's about our freedom; it's about the world we are leaving to our children, and to our grandchildren. The future of humanity is at stake.

We must get our message across. We must tell the world early treatment is the way forward. We must encourage doctors everywhere to embrace early treatment. We must tell the people, we must tell everyone, whether they are vaccinated or not, that they absolutely must seek early treatment if they are infected with COVID.

We need to tell the truth about COVID. We need to dispel the fear. We must be relentless in our efforts to tell the truth.

We must be united. And together, my friends, we will prevail.

This is my message to you, my fellow doctors and professionals, my friends. And this is also my message to the world.

My name is George Fareed. I am just a seventy-seven-year-old family doctor from Southern California, and I thank you for your attention.

After these introductory remarks at the summit, I also provided a testimony, similar to that from the November Senate hearings. However, I did add some additional recommendations:

If I were "king for a day," based on the science, the evidence in the literature, and my experience, I would propose the following approach to the pandemic:

- *The emphasis must be on early diagnosis and early treatment.*
- *Establish a massive education program for patients and doctors for early diagnosis of COVID.*
- *Everyone needs to know treatment works best if it is initiated in the first five to seven days.*
- *Establish community clinics for public access to early treatment of symptomatic COVID-19 infections.*

- *Educate primary care providers on the outpatient treatment protocol for symptomatic COVID-19 infections.*
- *No jurisdiction (local, state, or federal) can lock down public schools, businesses, places of worship, etc. With early treatment, there is no reason to shut down.*
- *High-risk health workers, high-risk teachers, and nursing home patients should take prophylaxis, especially during periods when there are high case numbers.*

After the historic Rome Summit concluded, I was recognized in the United States for my accomplishments in the Imperial Valley for my work with colleague Dr. Tyson in stemming the pandemic.

The following is excerpted from an article, "The Most Courageous Physician," published in *The Desert Review* on September 20, 2021:

> *Dr. Fareed's early cocktail employed a combination of hydroxychloroquine, azithromycin, and nutraceuticals, including zinc, vitamin D, and C. He explained this in his remarks in Rome,*
>
> *"Eighteen months ago, in March 2020, I, along with my colleague Dr. Brian Tyson, began treating COVID-19 patients early in the course of the disease with a combination of medications, initially primarily hydroxychloroquine and azithromycin or doxycycline, and nutraceuticals including zinc, vitamin D and C.*
>
> *"As Dr. McCullough explained, medications such as hydroxychloroquine act as ionophores to allow zinc into the cell to interfere with viral replication.*
>
> *"As time progressed, so did our treatment, and we added drugs such as Ivermectin, fluvoxamine, and monoclonal antibodies, as well as aspirin and budesonide (steroid) to treat the other aspects of the disease."*
>
> *To put Dr. Fareed's results in perspective, his county, Imperial, located in Southern California, has experienced 30,000 total COVID-19*

cases and 750 deaths. Drs. Fareed and Tyson treated over 20 percent of them, some 7,000 patients, and simple mathematics would have predicted their group would have had their share, or 150, of these deaths. Arguably they had one casualty.

Thus, they saved at least 149 patients or 99 percent with their protocol. Had the United States adopted it when Dr. Fareed advised the United States Senate on November 19, 2020, we could have saved 500,000 of the 650,000 deaths that occurred after his announcement.

As Dr. Fareed put it,

"This is a time that calls on the greatest of human attributes—courage. Everyone here must understand that we are in the greatest fight of our lives—when doctors are prevented from treating their patients with life-saving medicine, we know that something sinister is going on."[36]

One of Dr. Fareed's great accomplishments was his participation in the presentation of the Rome Physician's Declaration. This document, not unlike the U.S. Declaration of Independence enumerated a set of injustices that required correction. These injustices included the forced "one size fits all" strategy of treatment, the censorship of physicians' open discourse, and the obstacles to a physician's practice of his Hippocratic Oath.

The Rome Declaration was reviewed in this article published by the Desert Review on October 4, 2021.

---

36   Hope, J. R. (2021, September 20). "The Ivermectin Deworming Hoax—Part III: Poison Control Exposed." *The Desert Review*. Retrieved November 22, 2021, from https://www.thedesertreview.com/the-ivermectin-deworming-hoax--part-iii-poison-control-exposed/article_a553b7f2-1a31-11ec-881a-a7df53e98d65.html.

An international alliance of physicians and medical scientists met in Rome, Italy between September 12 and 14 for a three-day Global COVID Summit to speak "truth to power about COVID pandemic research and treatment." The summit presented an opportunity for the medical professionals to compare studies and assess the efficacy of the various treatments for the Coronavirus that have been developed in hospitals, doctors' offices, and research labs throughout the world.

However, many of these medical professionals have experienced career threats, character assassination, censorship of research papers, clinical trials, and patient observations, their professional history and accomplishments altered or omitted in academic and mainstream media because of them providing life-saving treatments for COVID patients.

Dr. Robert Malone, who discovered in-vitro and in-vivo RNA transfection and invented mRNA vaccines while he was at the Salk Institute in 1988, read the Declaration at the summit.

The Physicians' Declaration states:

We the physicians of the world, united and loyal to the Hippocratic Oath, recognizing the profession of medicine as we know it is at a crossroad, are compelled to declare the following;

WHEREAS, it is our utmost responsibility and duty to uphold and restore the dignity, integrity, art and science of medicine;

WHEREAS, there is an unprecedented assault on our ability to care for our patients;

WHEREAS, public policy makers have chosen to force a "one size fits all" treatment strategy, resulting in needless illness and death, rather than upholding fundamental concepts of the individualized, personalized approach to patient care which is proven to be safe and more effective;

WHEREAS, physicians and other health care providers working on the front lines, utilizing their knowledge of epidemiology, pathophysiology and pharmacology, are often first to identify new, potentially life-saving treatments;

WHEREAS, physicians are increasingly being discouraged from engaging in open professional discourse and the exchange of ideas about new and emerging diseases, not only endangering the essence of the medical profession, but more importantly, more tragically, the lives of our patients;

WHEREAS, thousands of physicians are being prevented from providing treatment to their patients, as a result of barriers put up by pharmacies, hospitals, and public health agencies, rendering the vast majority of healthcare providers helpless to protect their patients in the face of disease. Physicians are now advising their patients to simply go home (allowing the virus to replicate) and return when their disease worsens, resulting in hundreds of thousands of unnecessary patient deaths, due to failure-to-treat;

WHEREAS, this is not medicine. This is not care. These policies may actually constitute crimes against humanity.

NOW THEREFORE, IT IS:

RESOLVED, that the physician-patient relationship must be restored. The very heart of medicine is this relationship, which *allows physicians to best understand their patients and their illnesses, to formulate treatments that give the best chance for success, while the patient is an active participant in their care.*

RESOLVED, that the political intrusion into the practice of medicine and the physician/patient relationship must end. *Physicians, and all health care providers, must be free to practice the art and science of medicine without fear of retribution, censorship, slander, or disciplinary action, including possible loss of licensure and hospital privileges, loss of insurance contracts and interference from government entities and organizations – which further prevent us from caring for patients in need. More than ever, the right and ability to exchange objective scientific findings, which further our understanding of disease, must be protected.*

RESOLVED, that physicians must defend their right to prescribe treatment, observing the tenet FIRST, DO NO HARM. Physicians shall not be restricted from prescribing safe and effective treatments. These restrictions continue to cause unnecessary sickness and death. The rights of patients, after being fully informed about the risks and benefits of each option, must be restored to receive those treatments.

RESOLVED, that we invite physicians of the world and all health care providers to join us in this noble cause as we endeavor to restore trust, integrity and professionalism to the practice of medicine.

RESOLVED, that we invite the scientists of the world, who are skilled in biomedical research and uphold the highest ethical and moral standards, to insist on their ability to conduct and publish objective, empirical research without fear of reprisal upon their careers, reputations and livelihoods.

RESOLVED, that we invite patients, who believe in the importance of the physician-patient relationship and the ability to be active participants in their care, to demand access to science-based medical care.

Liberty Counsel Founder and Chairman Mat Staver said, "These medical professionals have been censored and threatened for simply upholding the Hippocratic Oath to 'do no harm.' Throughout history, many breakthrough discoveries that have now become accepted science were initially censored. It's past time to end medical censorship and allow doctors and scientific experts the freedom they rightfully deserve."

The Rome Summit and its Physicians' Declaration can be viewed as the culmination of Dr. Fareed's ground-breaking work with Dr. Tyson in the COVID-19 Pandemic. When many doctors would be content with remaining silent and not rocking the boat, Dr. Fareed decided to speak out against the most powerful forces in medicine, and he saved nearly ten thousand lives.

The Rome Physician's Declaration was signed by nearly 12,000 physicians and scientists worldwide at the time of this writing. We pray that it changes the way Pandemics are managed in the future and ensures that patient rights and a physician's Hippocratic Oath remain fundamental.[37]

---

37 "Thousands of medical professionals declare COVID policies 'Crimes Against Humanity.'" (2021, October 04). *The Desert Review*. Retrieved from https://www.thedesertreview.com/news/thousands-of-medical-professionals-declare-covid-policies-crimes-against-humanity/article_e2863f70-2074-11ec-8212-abe09d13e222.html.

CHAPTER 7

A NATIONAL COVID PLAN

One of the questions that comes up in the discussion of COVID-19 is regarding a national plan. While our elected leaders are not physicians, they are being challenged to present a plan for the country going forward. Considering that this is a medical issue, it logically follows that doctors are in the best position to articulate an approach that would address not only the virus, but also issues surrounding how best to resume our lives.

In September of 2020, three months before the roll-out of the vaccine, along with Dr. Donald Pompan, an orthopedic surgeon, and Dr. Michael Jacobs, a family medicine doctor with the Veterans Administration, we have crafted a national plan for COVID-19 that addresses both medical and societal concerns:

OUR NATIONAL PLAN FOR COVID-19:

- Protect the vulnerable (e.g., nursing home residents, elderly, those with chronic illnesses).
- No jurisdiction (local, state, or federal) can lock down public schools, businesses, places of worship, etc.
- Low virulence and morbidity in children and young adults preclude mass isolation and lockdowns of public schools and college campuses. Campus support staff can wear PPE and have confidence in prophylaxis and/or rapid treatment for concerning symptoms.
- Diagnosis of COVID-19 is based on symptoms with confirmatory testing after initiating treatment with the HCQ cocktail, especially for high-risk patients.
- Emphasis on outpatient treatment initiated immediately on high-risk patients based on well-established characteristic symptoms.
- Treatment with HCQ and ivermectin in the COVID-19 cocktail is most effective when prescribed within the first five days of symptoms. These medications may best be used along with the COVID-19 monoclonal antibody infusion given once. Additional anti-COVID-19 medications such as Fluvoxamine and those being reviewed by the FDA may enhance the efficacy of the treatment in analogy with the use of multiple antivirals with different mechanisms of action in the treatment of HIV and hepatitis C infections.
- Disrupt viral replication with the HCQ and ivermectin COVID-19 cocktail to prevent disease progression, hospitalization, and consumption of human and material resources.
- Establish community clinics for public access to early treatment of symptomatic COVID-19 infections.

- Form a massive education program to emphasize early diagnosis and treatment, independent of test results.
- Provide federal fiscal support for outpatient treatment of symptomatic COVID-19 patients.
- Educate primary care providers on the outpatient treatment protocol for symptomatic COVID-19 infections.
- Vulnerable teachers can wear PPE, use prophylaxis, or provide distant teaching options.
- Online schooling is an option for those unable to participate in in-person learning.
- Vulnerable individuals need to exercise caution with attendance at public events.
- Fever clinics should be set up in hotspots of infections and used for early diagnosis and treatment.[38]

This plan was introduced three months before having the vaccine. The only change we would have made to this protocol as time progressed was to have used the vaccine in high-risk groups such as the elderly and individuals with co-morbidities. Our plan would have reduced deaths through early treatment, protected the elderly initially by isolating them and later with vaccination, allowed businesses and schools to remain open, and society to go back to normal.

Unfortunately, our plan was not followed; our nation under the leadership of Dr. Fauci adopted a strategy of "hiding" from the virus until the vaccine was available. Then, when the vaccine failed to stop

---

38 Fareed, G. C. (2021, April 16). "Doctors pen National Plan for SARS-CoV-2/COVID-19." *The Desert Review.* Retrieved November 21, 2021, from https://www.thedesertreview.com/news/doctors-pen-national-plan-for-sars-cov-2-covid-19/article_6cee85fc-ee06-11ea-a631-23f68081bba0.html.

the spread, we hid again, relying on masks and social distancing while rejecting the one answer to ending the pandemic: early diagnosis and treatment.

Instead of following the mainstream "wait and see" approach, our plan would have kept people alive, and avoided traumatic and invasive measures like mass lockdowns. Our commonsense plan, which includes the use of the C19 protocol, is a game-changer in the national approach to COVID-19 morbidity and outcomes. Early treatment with the HCQ cocktail would have permitted our society to resume a semblance of normalcy and economic vitality.

Instead, our country embraced an approach driven by fear and not by science, and the results have been catastrophic with almost 800,000 dead (as of December 2021) and the economy in a tailspin. Most significantly, children were kept out of school. We took the exact opposite approach that we should have taken—the healthy never should have locked down.

This safe and effective outpatient treatment for COVID-19 will reduce disruptive and destructive fear. There would be no rationale to shut down schools. It would allow children to conduct themselves normally, and teachers with high-risk morbidities would be able to protect themselves with PPE and (if desired), even take the medication prophylactically.

Indeed, the plan that we proposed in September 2020, the cornerstone that is early treatment, is still relevant today; parents will be more comfortable sending their children to school, knowing a readily available outpatient treatment exists if their child were to develop a symptomatic COVID-19 infection. The recurring theme is to protect the most vulnerable while allowing the rest of society to get on with their lives.

There is no compelling reason to ever shut down a business again given that safe, effective treatments were readily available for high-risk individuals who develop symptomatic COVID-19 infections. There should never again be a lockdown, no matter what the next variant may be.

Our healthcare systems' agonizing predicament is the result of an abject failure to acknowledge and implement an existing safe and effective outpatient treatment protocol for symptomatic infections.

As far as testing, in most cases, it makes little sense to obtain a COVID-19 test unless one is going to do something with the result. A test can be negative one day and positive the next. It is not practical to test individuals daily. However, high-risk individuals (older than sixty and those with comorbidities) with well-recognized COVID-19 symptoms *can* be treated as early as possible with the hydroxychloroquine cocktail. A confirmatory test can be obtained prior to treatment (without waiting for the result), as the test outcome should not alter the minimal duration of the HCQ cocktail, which can be as short as five days.

A safe, effective outpatient treatment fosters a renewed focus on good judgment and best public-health practices (hand washing and social distancing), especially for the elderly and those with comorbidities. Masks may be helpful when indoors, in close proximity to others, as well. A safe, effective, accessible, evidence-based, science-based solution exists that can inspire confidence and mitigate fear.

The former FDA Director, Dr. Stephen Hahn, was, we believe, the principal obstacle to the implementation of a hydroxychloroquine-based outpatient treatment, falsely labeling the drug as "dangerous." Moreover, Dr. Fauci falsely characterized hydroxychloroquine as "ineffective." Please remember, merely designating someone an "expert" does not render Dr. Fauci's (or Dr. Hahn's) declarations infallible—especially considering the fact that nobody has scrutinized many of these opinions, which are not even supported by scientific evidence. Drs. Hahn and Fauci's falsehoods must be confronted and dismantled. Therefore, it is incumbent on our national medical leadership to implement outpatient treatment with the HCQ cocktail as an evidence-based, best-practices approach to the SARS-CoV-2/COVID-19 pandemic.

AN INVITATION

It is our sincere hope that you have found the information in this book to be informative and eye-opening. In fact, we hope you will consider joining us in the fight to get the word out about our national plan, as well as the scientifically sound information contained within these pages. Share what you are learning with friends and family; post information that challenges the mainstream media on your own social media accounts; reach out to your elected officials; read the studies referenced in this book and share the information with everyone you know!

When you become part of the solution, you will serve as an inspiration to a world that has been running in fear for far too long. We know that hope is already here, and it's ours for the taking—if we can work together as a unified country, educated, and prepared to overcome COVID, we can return to normalcy . . . normalcy that we desperately want, need, and *deserve*.

CHAPTER 8

OUR STATISTICAL RESEARCH SUMMARY

By Mathew Crawford

Mathew Crawford is an applied statistician who has worked in the actuarial field, as a quantitative trader on and off Wall Street. He has also written several textbook, is an educator, entrepreneur, and writer at www.roundingtheearth.substack.com.

Note: This chapter explains and reviews our research into the validity of early treatment for COVID and provides a scientific basis that confirms what we have seen and continue to see experientially in our approach to treating COVID. Provided is both the study itself and a detailed analysis of the study rational and outcomes.

"Such an action cannot be obtained by the process of choice or deliberation. To be effective, propaganda must constantly short-circuit all thought and decision. It must operate on the individual at the level of the unconscious. He must not know that he is being

shaped by outside forces (this is one of the conditions for the success of propaganda), but some central core in him must be reached in order to release the mechanism in the unconscious which will provide the appropriate—and expected—action."

—*Jacques Ellul, The Formation of Men's Attitudes*

In late April 2021, Dr. Brian Tyson contacted me and asked if I would be willing to run an analysis on the patient data that he had collected at the All Valley Urgent Care (AVUC) clinics he runs with the help of Dr. George Fareed. I had been watching interviews by the two physicians for months, and sharing their summary results with friends and social media communities within larger spreadsheets where I organized hydroxychloroquine early treatment data from around the world. At my newsletter, roundingtheearth.substack.com, I had written about the need to examine and compare data at a protocol level,[39] meaning a comparison not simply of who received what drug or medical care, but the entire procedural framework of medical care. In particular, this includes aspects of treatment such as how quickly the process of medical care began over the course of viral infection of illness. Dr. Tyson agreed that we should conduct the analysis in a matter that distinguishes early treatment results from late treatment results.

The invitation to collaborate on this research was a great honor to me. It was also an opportunity to put my hands on data that would help me better understand the strange insanity I thought I was seeing in

---

39 Crawford, M. (2021, April 2). "The Chloroquine Wars Part IX: How to Rig Research by Statistically Stacking the Deck (A Simpson's Paradox Tale)." Retrieved December 7, 2021, from https://roundingtheearth.substack.com/p/the-chloroquine-wars-part-ix.

the projected media image of the medical community, not to mention attitudes among some of my personal friends that made talking about the key statistics difficult. By this time, I had been served two thirty-day suspensions from Facebook for violating "Community Standards" talking about my communications with doctors and researchers in India who supported the use of hydroxychloroquine and ivermectin in preventing SARS-CoV-2 infection and in treating COVID-19.

These admonitions from social media fact-checkers for the crime of reporting on medical conversations pushed me to want to do more, hence my budding Substack newsletter and commitment to the AVUC data project. I was in search of ways to help sort out the unnecessary aspects of all the pandemonium. Prior to communication with Dr. Tyson, my own data gathering included results from researchers and physicians around the world, including

- Dr. Didier Raoult[40] (the world's most well-published communicable disease expert[41]) and his colleagues in France;
- Dr. Vipul Shah, who helped mold India's COVID-19 treatment protocol for other doctors and healthcare workers;
- Dr. Vladimir Zelenko in New York, USA;
- Dr. Luigi Cavanna in Italy, who started taking hydroxychloroquine to patients outside overflowing Italian hospitals so that *none* of them died and few needed hospitalization;
- Dr. Brian Armstrong and Dr. Brian Procter in Texas, USA;

40 Raoult, D. (November 2, 2020). Curriculum Vitae. Retrieved December 7, 2021, from https://www.mediterranee-infection.com/wp-content/uploads/2020/11/CV-Didier-RAOULT-nov2020.pdf.
41 Expertscape. "Expertise in Communicable Diseases: Worldwide." Retrieved December 7, 2021, from https://web.archive.org/web/20200327083328/https://expertscape.com/ex/communicable+diseases.

- The physicians staffing 238 outpatient clinics in Saudi Arabia[42];
- and numerous others.

As best as I could tell, their patients suffered around 98% lower mortality than others in their same geographic regions. Dr. Tyson told me that patients going through his protocol at AVUC suffered a 0.07% mortality rate (one death per 1,500 or so COVID-19 cases) while the mortality rate in Imperial County, California, where the clinics were located, was over 3% (1 death per 33 COVID-19 cases), right in line with my 98% estimate.

Over the months, I had wondered to myself if *anyone* really had to die from COVID-19. Maybe that handful of deaths among patients receiving all three of hydroxychloroquine, azithromycin, and zinc supplementation were simply people who would have died, regardless. After all, the bulk of COVID-19 fatalities was among the very elderly, with an average age in the high seventies in the United States, and over eighty in many Western nations.[43]

How could any caring person in leadership fail to recognize such dramatic differentials in treatment statistics? How could it be that my aggregated data of over ten thousand patients drifted between a 0.05 to 0.09% case fatality rate (proportion deceased) from COVID-19 while every day the press gave Dr. Anthony Fauci a forum and essentially zero pushback when he repeatedly denigrated such results as "anecdotal."

---

42   Mohana, Abdulrhman et al. "Hydroxychloroquine Safety Outcome within Approved Therapeutic Protocol for COVID-19 Outpatients in Saudi Arabia." *International journal of infectious diseases : IJID : official publication of the International Society for Infectious Diseases* vol. 102 (2021): 110-114. doi:10.1016/j.ijid.2020.10.031

43   Swiss Policy Research. (May 2020, updated November 2021). "Studies on Covid-19 Lethality." Retrieved December 7, 2021, from https://swprs.org/studies-on-covid-19-lethality/#3-median-age-of-covid-19-deaths-per-country.

Isn't the way to turn anecdotes into data to collect, verify, and aggregate them? Wouldn't it be great if there existed something like a public health institution tasked with doing that?

Within a few days, I received Dr. Tyson's data and went to work. The initial process of cleaning and organizing the AVUC data took two full weeks. Writing the paper took another week. Though we have made some minor edits since, the following is the text of our still unpublished research on patients treated with the AVUC COVID-19 protocols between March 1, 2020, and March 31, 2021. Some readers may want to skip reading the paper but may want to look at the summary tables presented at the end of the paper. After all, scientific papers are generally inaccessible to lay people, and it takes time to learn to read them well.

However, readers with some understanding of statistics may find some aspects of the paper interesting. After the paper, I will discuss some aspects of the analysis, and a few things that went wrong in science and medicine in particular that contributed to the delayed publication of this and likely many other data series. I will do my best to keep statistical and scientific jargon to a minimum and explain the terms where I use them. Such research as follows would have ended the primary pain of the pandemic during its first few months if broadly gathered. Consider this as you examine the data summary.

Low Rates of Hospitalization and Death in 4,376 COVID-19 Patients Given Early Ambulatory Medical and Supportive Care.

A Case Series and Observational Study.

Contributors to the study:

Brian M. Tyson, M.D., George Fareed, M.D., Emmanuel Beltran Guiterrez, M.D., Robert Villegas, NP, Edgar Josue Anaya Gomez, M.D., Paloma Serrano Lopez, M.D., Ernesto Breton Herrera, M.D., Jesus Palomera III, M.D., Christiany Alexandrah Morales, Ana Mariella Escutia Gonzalez, Fabiola Tyson, NP, M.D., Mathew Crawford

Address for Correspondence
Mathew Crawford
mathew.crawford@protonmail.com

Word Count: 4046
Funding source(s): self-funded
Conflict of interest statement for author: nothing to disclose
Authors had access to the data and wrote the manuscript
Running head: Outcomes after Ambulatory Treatment of COVID-19

Abstract

Background: This study reports the results of early ambulatory protocols in treating 4,376 COVID-19 patients at All Valley Urgent Care (AVUC) facilities in Imperial County, CA, and compares those treatment results to outcomes of other patients in the same county during a nearly identical time period, and encourages a better framework for analysis of such results while adding to the growing body of evidence as to whether such treatment reduces the need for hospitalization and lowers mortality rates. The broad application of face-to-face ambulatory treatment of SARS-CoV-2 infection has not broadly been undertaken in the United States.

Methods: We examine the results of two similar multidrug protocols with data from the immediate county. Protocol 1 uses of hydroxychloroquine, an agent with apparent antiviral reactivity against SARS-CoV-2, two antibiotics (azithromycin, doxycycline), along with a multivitamin pack (including zinc, vitamin C, vitamin D, and others), and with selective use of one or a combination of inhaled budesonide, dexamethasone, prednisone, or other treatments deemed appropriate. Protocol 2 includes all of these options, plus ivermectin where deemed appropriate by physicians. Results were then stratified according to disease severity of patients when first seen by doctors. Among 4,385 individuals sorted in both protocols and three severity levels, combined or excluded from this study, the mean age was 40.5 ± 18.2 years and 12.8% were greater than twenty years of age.

Primary Results: Among 3,962 patients treated for mild COVID-19, prior to the development of moderate or severe levels of disease stage, none died as compared to 3.03% (2.25% risk adjusted) (OR = 0.0000, $p < 0.0001$) in the same county and time period. Of those 3,962 patients, 0.05% were hospitalized as compared to 22.68% (20.76% risk adjusted) (OR = 0.0019, $p < 0.0001$) in the same county and time period. Differences in outcomes among All Valley Urgent Care patients based on the severity at the time of presentation were observed. Those patients receiving treatment while presenting mild COVID-19 were less often hospitalized (OR = 0.0293, $p < 0.0001$) and suffered lower mortality (OR = 0.0000, p = 0.0008). Results suggest a highly significant impact for these multidrug protocols. No serious side effects, including cardiac side effects, were observed.

Key words: SARS-CoV-2; COVID-19; multidrug; hospitalization; mortality; ambulatory; antiviral; zinc; hydroxychloroquine; ivermectin; doxycycline; azithromycin; vitamin; corticosteroid

1. Introduction

The epidemic viral outbreak of SARS-CoV-2 infection (COVID-19) still persists across the United States as mass vaccination is attempted using technologies new and old, without any publicly demonstrated cost-benefit analysis, lingering questions about short- and long-term safety both, and perhaps too late in the pandemic to achieve optimal results.[1] There are still no approved drugs or drug combinations in the U.S. indicated for the ambulatory treatment of COVID-19 or its complications.

Unfortunately, there are no potentially conclusive randomized trials of early ambulatory multidrug therapy underway at this time. While some medical researchers announced promising treatments very early during the pandemic[2, 3]—often multidrug therapeutic protocols administered as early as possible upon symptoms[4]—little attention has been paid to such results by the FDA or any other similar Western medical bodies.[5] In particular, there are now numerous studies indicating the efficacy of hydroxychloroquine (HCQ) and ivermectin (IVM) in outpatient treatment or for mild COVID-19 patients who could be served by early ambulatory care.[6, 7]

Doctors at All Valley Urgent Care (AVUC)—as well as others in the U.S. and around the world—used hydroxychloroquine within outpatient treatment protocols, providing the rationale for treatments examined in this paper. Later, ivermectin was added as a nearly uniformly positive body of evidence of its apparent efficacy was reported.[8] Still, there is a vast pool of often uncollected or unpublished data regarding these treatments (personal correspondences).

As with all serious medical conditions, there is a role for empiric treatment in an attempt to reduce fatalities.[9] This study provides a report that updates the totality of real-world data regarding multidrug protocols for the ambulatory care of a substantial number of patients with mild COVID-19, prior to progression to moderate or severe COVID-19 conditions.

We further summarize the logic behind emphasizing data within a picture of treatment optimization as opposed to a hierarchy of methodological preferences not tailored to the task. When waiting means losing lives to illness, rapid experimentation with safe, low-cost treatments is practical, economic science on a level that every physician can employ. Indeed, it is their ethical duty.

Risk stratification and advised nutraceuticals were in line with previously published guidance,[10] although physicians were allowed to exercise judgment. For instance, hydroxychloroquine or ivermectin were prescribed to patients deemed high risk who were PCR-positive prior to the development of any symptoms. All patients received empiric treatment on the first day of presentation in most cases before COVID-19 test results and treatment was continued for those with confirmed COVID-19. The protocols utilized agents with antiviral activity against SARS-CoV-2 (zinc, hydroxychloroquine, ivermectin) and one antibiotic (azithromycin, doxycycline, ceftriaxone), along with inhaled budesonide and/or intramuscular dexamethasone.

Albuterol nebulizer, inhaled budesonide, intravenous volume expansion with supplemental parenteral thiamine 500 mg, magnesium sulfate 4 grams, folic acid 1 gram, and vitamin B12 1 mg were administered for severely ill patients who either present or return to the clinic with severe symptoms.[11] Additionally, for the severely ill population, dexamethasone 8 mg and ceftriaxone 1 gram was administered intramuscularly. A total of eight patients received monoclonal antibody treatment. All patients had in-person or telemedicine follow up at forty-eight hours, and as needed, depending on the duration and intensity of symptoms.[12]

Hospitalization and death data were collected on follow-up telemedicine visits or calls to family members. For the purpose of this paper, patients treated through October 21, 2020, were treated within Protocol 1, which includes all options listed above excluding ivermectin, and those treated October 22, 2020, through March 31, 2021, were treated within Protocol 2, which added ivermectin as an option.

[The paper includes a protocol chart that is Figure 3 in McCullough et al in Reviews in Cardiovascular Medicine: https://rcm.imrpress.com/article/2020/2153-8174/RCM2020264.shtml]

2. Methods

2.1 Setting

Here, we report clinical outcomes associated with empiric multidrug regimens for confirmed COVID-19 patients who present to All Valley Urgent Care, which is a large, dedicated SARS-CoV-2 treatment center in El Centro, CA, between (Protocol 1) January 12, 2020, and October 21, 2020, and also (Protocol 2) between October 22, 2020, and March 13, 2021, endpoints inclusive. We compare the outcomes of the patients to which these protocols were applied against all 20,921 other known COVID-19 cases within Imperial County, CA during a similar time period (through May 3, 2021) where All Valley Urgent Care is located. Calculations for comparisons between groups and subgroups were performed using Excel or GraphPad Prism. Patient data for both All Valley Urgent Care and for Imperial County, CA was verified as received by the Public Health Department of Imperial County.

2.2 Inclusion-Exclusion and Categorization Criteria

Of the 4,385 COVID-19 patients recorded by Valley Urgent Care, a total of 3,962 treated patients were deemed to suffer from mild COVID-19 upon presentation, while 414 treated, but not immediately hospitalized patients had already progressed to moderate or severe COVID-19 stages of illness. One of those patients was treated for severe COVID-19, refusing immediate hospitalization. A total of nine patients were excluded due to nontreatment either because they were immediately sent to a hospital or because they refused treatment.

2.3 Confirmation of COVID-19 Diagnosis

Prior to May 15, 2020, patients were diagnosed with COVID-19 based on antibody-positive tests and symptom presentation per standard case definition guidance. From May 15, 2020, onward, patients underwent and tested positive using contemporary real-time polymerase chain reaction (PCR) assay tests from anterior nasal swab samples.

2.4 Patients

Among the 4,376 patients treated by All Valley Urgent Care staff, 2,137 (48.8%) were male, 2,239 (51.2%) were female, and 1,391 (31.8%) were fifty or older. Among these patients were 1,370 (31.3%) asymptomatic at presentation. A total of 1,980 (45.2%) patients received hydroxychloroquine, a total of 365 (8.3%) received ivermectin, while a total of 347 (7.9%) received both hydroxychloroquine and ivermectin.

2.5 Protocol Rationale

Prior to the COVID-19 pandemic, researchers noted the numerous general and specific qualities suggesting hydroxychloroquine's potential to treat future coronavirus outbreaks.[13-16] Shortly after the emergence of SARS-CoV-2, South Korea,[17] and China[18] rushed to a recommendation of hydroxychloroquine usage and a standard of care of the highly similar chloroquine drug in particular. Multiple rationale papers encouraged the research and medical communities to examine the effects of hydroxychloroquine.[19-21]

As hydroxychloroquine began to be used for prophylaxis or early ambulatory treatment in many nations such as India[22, 23] and Italy,[24] it is noteworthy that its use grew in popularity rather than shrank. There seem to be no stories at all of doctors abandoning the use of hydroxychloroquine in outpatient care in the practice of empiric medicine, except where prohibited. This observation should not be viewed simply as evidence, but strong enough evidence to make it a priority for public health authorities to make it a commitment to turn anecdotes into working data.

Additionally, scores of studies have examined results from the use of hydroxychloroquine either as monotherapy or in multidrug regimens, as treatment for COVID-19 patients (listed at https://c19hcq.com/). We first note that many more of these studies reported more favorable results among patients receiving hydroxychloroquine, including conclusions in both categories (monotherapy or in a multidrug regimen) that did or did not reach statistical significance in isolation.[25] While one such study can conceivably ascertain a high likelihood of causal reduction of disease progression or mortality through traditional tools of inferential statistics, some have claimed to demonstrate a lack of efficacy or even harm resulting from the use of hydroxychloroquine.

The latter form of conclusion results *prima facia* from the fallacy of assuming no other protocols exist that could improve the performance of the applied treatment. In fact, in fourteen out of fourteen published studies examining the mortality results of early treatment (largely at the mild stage prior to moderate disease progression) of COVID-19 patients with a moderate dose of hydroxychloroquine (no higher than 6g in total, but usually between 1.6g and 4.0g, spread out over several days), the treatment arm suffered lower mortality than the control arm.[25] Logically, the success of any one treatment protocol represents the success of the medications used in that protocol. For instance, the results in Figure 1 represent a successful outcome, given a sufficiently powered sample size.

Further, there seems to be little if any effort to review the body of literature of the application of hydroxychloroquine, ivermectin, and other potentially effective therapeutics with the goal of *optimizing* outcomes that would, in a virtuous cycle, necessarily further tilt the summary of effects toward even greater efficacy of multidrug regimens

The Hydrocychloroquine Hypothesis

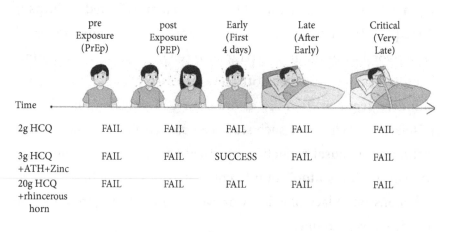

	pre Exposure (PrEp)	post Exposure (PEP)	Early (First 4 days)	Late (After Early)	Critical (Very Late)
Time					
2g HCQ	FAIL	FAIL	FAIL	FAIL	FAIL
3g HCQ +ATH+Zinc	FAIL	FAIL	SUCCESS	FAIL	FAIL
20g HCQ +rhincerous horn	FAIL	FAIL	FAIL	FAIL	FAIL

Figure 1

such as the protocols we analyze in this study. By denying the value of empiric evidence and the experience of the doctors applying early ambulatory protocols to patients, health authorities miss the opportunity to collect valuable data and help those and other doctors network to share life-saving observations.

2.6 Analysis of Patient Outcomes by Protocol, Time Dependence, and Aggregation

The examination of the efficacy of potential antiviral agents requires progression-dependent stratification of results since antiviral effects are largest prior to the maturity of the viral replication process. For an antiviral drug effective in the treatment of COVID-19, results of patients treated early, at the mild disease state should be categorically different from the results of patients treated at the moderate disease stage, which may be further distinct from the results of patients treated after the onset of severe COVID-19.

Aggregating the results of treatments of a potential antiviral agent can dramatically alter effect sizes, and even produce results Simpson's paradoxes (or more generally "Simpson's effects" where data trends may not reverse, but appear dampened in magnitude), making effective treatments appear less helpful or even harmful. The skew in effect results after aggregation of patients of differing viral progression for an effective antiviral is clearly monotonic and negative, obscuring or reverse quantified effects.

The following hypothetical, but realistic charts demonstrate the need for stratification of results. In our hypothetical, the drug XYZ is assumed to reduce mortality by 60% when given to patients upon reaching Severity Score 4 of the WHO's ordinal scale, as we see in direct protocol-level comparisons of Hospitals 1 and 3. However, a naïve analysis comparing patients who received drug XYZ to those who did not would conclude that drug XYZ results in a 37% relative *increase* in mortality, as demonstrated shown in Figure 2.

Often, studies attempt to correct such analysis in insufficient ways. For instance, grouping Hospitals 1 and 2 (those that use drug XYZ) against Hospital 3 would show a 40% reduction in mortality as opposed to the full 60% reduction in mortality.

Further, note that nothing in this hypothetical analysis implies anything about the efficacy of drug XYZ when given to patients earlier than at the point of hospitalization as should be optimal if drug XYZ has antiviral effects. There is no reason why, or any information that contradicts the possibility that drug XYZ, which seemed to do more harm than good in the original hypothetical analysis, could not effectively cure 100% of patients when applied very early. In particular,

COVID-19 Severity	Hospital 1 Drug XYZ Treatment for all cases		Hospital 2 Drug XYZ Treatment for all cases only		Hospital 3 No Treatment	
	Patients Progressing to Each Stage		Patients Progressing to Each Stage		Patients Progressing to Each Stage	
	Number	Percent(%)	Number	Percent(%)	Number	Percent(%)
4	1000	100%	1000	100%	1000	100%
5	500	50%	850	85%	850	85%
6	240	24%	400	40%	400	40%
7	120	12%	200	20%	250	25%
8	60	6%	120	12%	150	15%
9	30	3%	80	8%	90	9%
10 (death)	20	2%	40	4%	50	5%

Analysis of Drug XYZ Mortality From All Three Hospitals

	XYZ Treatment	NO XYZ Treatment
# of Patients	1400	1600
# Deceased	60	50
Mortality Rate	4.3%	3.1%

Figure 2

such results would still be consistent with an antiviral agent. While statisticians run results through Bayesian rubrics designed to correct for such flaws, such corrections may or may not come close to a perfect correction since, as we demonstrated, true optimal efficacy can still range anywhere from 60% to 100%. Stratifying results according to patient severity prevents these unnecessary flaws in the analysis.

Further, we suggest that much of the COVID-19 literature, most specifically that which examines effects of hydroxychloroquine as treatment, undergo re-analysis under a framework that separates analysis by protocol (specifically including severity stage at the time of treatment) rather than by sorting patients into binary categories defined by whether or not they received a particular drug without (enough) respect for the overall protocol. We also recommend that meta-analyses of hydroxychloroquine treatment results discontinue the inclusion of all studies that do not distinguish results at the protocol level, including stratification by the timing of treatment, and that studies included in such analyses necessarily be grouped according to stages of COVID-19 at which point treatment is delivered to each patient.

As we have heard the phrase, "garbage in, garbage out" applied to meta-analyses, so too should we apply it to studies such as the SOLIDARITY trials,[26] and other randomized control trials' (RCTs) use of hydroxychloroquine as monotherapy in exceptionally high and potentially dangerous doses on late-stage patients.[27] Any conclusion that such an RCT could demonstrate the lack of efficacy of hydroxychloroquine in other protocols is non-sequitur and demonstrates that basic logic and critical thinking are, and have always been, the true gold standards of science.

Finally, we note that the form of retrospective observational analysis we present in this paper generates results nearly identical in nature and value to those of RCTs (using similar protocols).[28, 29] While it is technically conceivable that some unknown confounding variable both sorts the patients visiting Valley Urgent Care clinics from those in the general population and also affects disease progression, most such bias is likely corrected by the demographic risk analysis we apply in the following results—particularly given the recognized importance of age as a variable in predicting outcomes, along with the substantial, if imperfect, correlation between age and primary comorbidities. Most unknown confounding variables would also likely have been observed and documented at this point in a pandemic.

The number of patients in this study is large enough to lower the variance inherent in random sorting of unexamined risk factors as a proportion of sample size, and the effect sizes observed in this analysis are extremely large. As sample sizes grow large, the observed results of observational studies and RCTs tend to converge.[28, 29]

2.7 Sensitivity Analysis

First and foremost, this study presents a large case series. We do our best to make the most of the results with comparison to both the local county case summary results, and synthetic versions of the county data. The primary limitation of our analysis is the synthetic comparator. In particular, nursing home patients who make up a substantial proportion of COVID-19 fatalities rarely overlap with patients seen at facilities such as ACUV. Our age mapping improves the comparison, but is still imperfect. In order to test the limitations, we compare the results of the treatment group to ideal cohorts under assumptions of varying hospitalization and mortality rates. The resulting confidence intervals suggest that even if imperfections in comparison warrant wider bounds, the resulting odds ratios are compelling.

3. Results

Given how few of the patients in Protocols 1 and 2 progressed to moderate or severe COVID-19, there was too little variation in results to confidently distinguish between the protocols on a statistical level, which could only be determined by extraordinarily large patient cohorts. This also means the positive results of this multidrug regimen can be more easily ascribed to hydroxychloroquine than to ivermectin, the primary hypothesized antiviral agents, though patients receiving ivermectin fared extremely well.

On the whole, the totality of effects can only be ascribed to the protocols as a whole, meaning there may be synergistic effects of some agents employed, or specific utility in the use of others (such as steroids). Each patient data set for Protocol 1, Protocol 2, and the combined patient aggregates showed dramatically lower rates of hospitalization and mortality relative to the general population in Imperial County, CA.

We note the limitations of retrospective observational studies with synthetic controls due to the lack of opportunity to sort at random or match them by propensity score, but believe that the glaringly small odds ratios, the combination of high patient numbers, and wide sensitivity analysis provide ample room for a declaration of significant positive results. Most certainly, the safety of numerous medications is demonstrated by the lack of serious adverse events for a substantial number of patients receiving each of hydroxychloroquine, ivermectin, azithromycin, doxycycline, albuterol, and budesonide.

The Valley Urgent care patient sets included fewer COVID-19 patients seventy or older (6.3%) than the larger county population (9.3%), and were more often male (48.8% vs. 47.4%). Mortality skewed heavily toward male COVID-19 sufferers in Imperial County. There is no way of knowing how many patients not treated at the Valley Urgent Care clinics also received similar forms of early ambulatory care including the medicines used in Protocols 1 and 2, so a comparison may result in dampened measures of relative risk for such outpatient treatment. Prior to computing p-values using Fisher's Exact Test, we corrected for age using mortality factors implicit in the county-wide data (excluding patients in our Protocol 1 and 2 groupings).

Among 20,921 COVID-19 patients in Imperial County, CA who were not treated by Valley Urgent Care, 4,770 (22.8%) were hospitalized and 636 died (3.0%).

Of 1,585 patients treated for mild COVID-19 in Protocol 1, there was one hospitalization (0.06%) and zero deaths (0%). Of 2,356 patients treated for mild COVID-19 in Protocol 2, there was one hospitalization (0.04%) and zero deaths (0%). There were twenty-one patients whose date of treatment was obscured after data blinding, but were treated for mild COVID-19, all without hospitalization or death. In total, of 3,962 patients (Table 1) treated for mild COVID-19 by All Valley Urgent Care staff, prior to moderate or severe disease progression, there were two hospitalizations (0.05%, RR = 0.0019, p < 0.0001) and zero deaths (0%, RR = 0.00, p < 0.0001).

Of 413 patients treated for moderate COVID-19 in Protocol 1, there were two hospitalizations (0.5%) and zero deaths (0%). Of 190 patients treated for moderate COVID-19 in Protocol 2, there were five hospitalizations (2.6%) and three deaths (1.6%). There was one patient treated whose date of treatment was obscured after data blinding, but was treated for moderate COVID-19 without hospitalization or death. In total, of 413 patients (Table 2) treated for moderate COVID-19 by Valley Urgent Care, there were seven hospitalizations (1.7%) and three deaths (OR = 0.0659, p < 0.0001). The one patient who refused hospitalization, and instead chose outpatient treatment for severe COVID-19 with All Valley Urgent Care recovered.

Those receiving treatment while presenting mild COVID-19 were less often hospitalized (OR = 0.0293, p < 0.0001) and suffered lower mortality (OR = 0.0000, p = 0.0008).

To understand the limitations of comparison, we ran a sensitivity analysis. Comparison groups included Imperial County's data through May 15, 2021, a version of that cohort with age profiles adjusted (corrected) to match the All Valley Urgent Care patient profiles, and several cohorts with decreasing hospitalization and mortality. Finally, we computed the lower bounds of hospitalization and mortality numbers for which the All Valley Urgent Care showed statistically significant improvement, which were a 0.20% hospitalization rate and a 0.10% case fatality rate (Table 3).

We note here that corrections for comorbidities or symptoms is both impossible and unnecessary for this analysis. It is impossible because such information is rarely gathered prior to the point of hospitalization, which is nearly always the demarcation point between mild and moderate COVID-19. These other factors are also highly correlated with age distribution, and with such a large sample size, it is doubtful that the data relationships change substantially.

4. Discussion

A handful of analyses have been published on early ambulatory care of COVID-19 patients. While almost uniformly positive with respect to hydroxychloroquine and ivermectin specifically, as well as smaller numbers of studies on fluvoxamine, proxalutamide, bromhexine, and other drugs, there is a vast amount of still uncollected data on these and numerous other treatments.

Such data collection should always have been a high priority for health officials and the larger medical community. It should have been a national priority. Going forward, it should be entirely unacceptable that any organization discourages the collection, organization, examination, and analysis of empiric treatment regimens developed by caring, diligent, and networked health professionals. To the extent that public health authorities operate, it should be inherent in their duties to encourage if not participate in that process as a primary duty.

We believe that that the case for early ambulatory care for COVID-19 patients utilizing multidrug regimens such as those described in this paper, using hydroxychloroquine, ivermectin, or potentially improvements on these options, has been amply demonstrated. The collection of unexamined pools of data, analyzed on a similar protocol level, will further demonstrate the case for early ambulatory treatment, and in particular, using multidrug regimens under similar or other protocols. Optimization of medical treatment cannot fully take place until these results are recognized, either by health officials, if not by the larger community of physicians capable of delivering these treatments or their patients.

It is difficult to imagine that optimization would involve the current standard of leaving patients untreated until the development of moderate or severe COVID-19 symptoms. All pertinent data suggests otherwise.

5. Conclusion

Our study found that early ambulatory treatment for SARS-CoV-2 infection and resulting COVID-19 disease is extremely safe, feasible, practical, and scalable to large numbers of patients. It is extremely important to encourage early ambulatory treatment, both among patients and doctors alike. These results demonstrate that hospitalization and death were nearly nonexistent when patients were treated with multidrug regimens in protocols that included hydroxychloroquine and ivermectin prior to progression beyond the mild COVID-19 disease state.

Similar therapies also showed statistically significant reductions in hospitalization and death among those treated during the moderate COVID-19 disease state. Given the depth of the COVID-19 crisis and the high mortality rate for hospital-initiated treatment, we conclude that early ambulatory multi-drug therapy should be a standard of care for high-risk patients. It is no longer tenable to delay treatment until a hospitalization for patients who can easily be treated early as outpatients with a well-managed protocol.

Acknowledgments

The authors thank all of the doctors and medical staff at the All Valley Urgent Care clinics, the Public Health Department of Imperial County, CA, as well as the maintainers of the Imperial County COVID-19 data and associated tracking systems. We thank all of the doctors and researchers who have thoughtfully generated so much useful research during the pandemic, and particularly those whose insights into early ambulatory treatment protocols encouraged the practice of valuable care at All Valley Urgent Care and this analysis of the data.

Funding

This study was entirely self-funded.

Competing Interests

None of the authors reports any conflicts of interest.

Table 1: AVUC Patients Presenting as Mild COVID-19

Prorocal 1

Age Range	Total N	Hospitalizations	Non-Survivors	Survivors	Hydroxychloroquine
0-9	42	0	0	42	2
10-19	136	0	0	136	13
20-29	322	0	0	322	64
30-39	329	0	0	329	81
40-49	290	0	0	290	60
50-59	266	0	0	266	83
60-69	129	1	0	129	41
70-79	60	0	0	60	21
80-89	10	0	0	10	2
90+	1	0	0	1	0
Total	1585	1	0	1585	367

Prorocal 2

Age Range	Total N	Hospitalizations	Non-Survivors	Survivors	Hydroxychloroquine	Ivermectin
0-9	90	0	0	90	0	0
10-19	280	0	0	280	39	12
20-29	393	0	0	393	202	46
30-39	495	0	0	495	288	49
40-49	389	0	0	389	245	52
50-59	320	0	0	320	196	51
60-69	237	0	0	237	162	61
70-79	110	1	0	110	85	24
80-89	39	0	0	39	25	5
90+	3	0	0	3	2	2
Total	2356	1	0	2356	1244	302

All Patients Treated for Mild COVID-19

Age Range	Total N	Hospitalizations	Non-Survivors	Survivors	Hydroxychloroquine	Ivermectin
0-9	132	0	0	132	2	0
10-19	418	0	0	418	52	12
20-29	722	0	0	722	266	46
30-39	828	0	0	828	369	49
40-49	682	0	0	682	305	52
50-59	587	0	0	587	279	51
60-69	368	1	0	368	203	61
70-79	172	1	0	172	106	24
80-89	49	0	0	49	27	5
90+	4	0	0	4	2	2
Total	3962	2	0	3962	1611	302

Table 2: AVUC Patients Presenting as Moderate COVID-19

Protocal 1

Age Range	Total N	Hospitalizations	Non-Survivors	Survivors	Hydroxychloroquine
0-9	1	0	0	1	0
10-19	2	0	0	2	2
20-29	28	0	0	28	22
30-39	35	0	0	35	31
40-49	58	1	0	58	53
50-59	46	1	0	46	42
60-69	32	0	0	32	29
70-79	13	0	0	13	12
80-89	7	0	0	7	6
90+		0	0	0	0
Total	222	2	0	222	197

Prorocal 2

Age Range	Total N	Hospitalizations	Non-Survivors	Survivors	Hydroxychloroquine	Ivermectin
0-9	1	0	0	1	0	0
10-19	5	0	0	5	2	1
20-29	16	0	0	16	13	8
30-39	23	0	0	23	21	7
40-49	33	1	0	33	29	12
50-59	41	1	1	40	38	15
60-69	42	2	2	40	40	12
70-79	22	0	0	22	22	6
80-89	6	1	0	6	6	2
90+	1	0	0	1	1	0
Total	190	5	3	187	172	63

All Patients Treated for Moderate COVID-19

Age Range	Total N	Hospitalizations	Non-Survivors	Survivors	Hydroxychloroquine	Ivermectin
0-9	2	0	0	2	0	0
10-19	7	0	0	7	4	12
20-29	44	0	0	44	35	46
30-39	58	0	0	58	52	49
40-49	92	2	0	92	82	52
50-59	87	2	1	86	80	51
60-69	74	2	2	72	69	61
70-79	35	0	0	35	34	24
80-89	13	1	0	13	12	5
90+	1	0	0	1	1	2
Total	413	7	3	410	369	302

Table 3	comparison of outcomes of patients to AVUC with mild COVID-19 (prior or further disease progression						
Hospitalized **Died**		Protocol 1 N = 1585 1 (0.06%) 0 (0.00%)		Protocol 2 N = 2356 1 (0.04%) 0 (0.00%)		All Patients N = 3962 2 (0.05%) 0 (0.00%)	
Imperial Country, CA Hospitalized Died	N = 20921 4,770 (22.80%) 636 (3.04%)	OR = 0.0021 OR = 0.0000	p < 0.0001 p < 0.0001	OR = 0.0014 OR = 0.0000	p < 0.0001 p < 0.0001	OR = 0.0017 OR = 0.0000	p < 0.0001 p < 0.0001
Imperial (Corrected) Hospitalized Died	N = 20921 4,343 (20.76%) 471 (2.25%)	OR = 0.0024 OR = 0.0000	p < 0.0001 p < 0.0001	OR = 0.0016 OR = 0.0000	p < 0.0001 p < 0.0001	OR = 0.0019 OR = 0.0000	p < 0.0001 p < 0.0001
Synethic 1 Hospitalized Died	N = 20921 3,138 (15.00%) 314 (1.50%)	OR = 0.0036 OR = 0.0000	p < 0.0001 p < 0.0001	OR = 0.0024 OR = 0.0000	p < 0.0001 p < 0.0001	OR = 0.0029 OR = 0.0000	p < 0.0001 p < 0.0001
Synethic 2 Hospitalized Died	N = 20921 2,092 (10.00%) 209 (1.00%)	OR = 0.057 OR = 0.0000	p < 0.0001 p < 0.0001	OR = 0.0038 OR = 0.0000	p < 0.0001 p < 0.0001	OR = 0.0045 OR = 0.0000	p < 0.0001 p < 0.0001
Synethic 3 Hospitalized Died	N = 20921 1,046 (5.00%) 105 (0.50%)	OR = 0.0120 OR = 0.0000	p < 0.0001 p < 0.0008	OR = 0.0080 OR = 0.0000	p < 0.0001 p < 0.0001	OR = 0.0096 OR = 0.0000	p < 0.0001 p < 0.0001
Limit of Significance Hospitalized Died	N = 20921 41 (0.20%) 21 (0.10%)					OR = 0.2572 OR = 0.0000	p < 0.0376 p < 0.0380

Bibliography for Study

1. McCullough PA, Eidt J, Rangaswami J, et al. "Urgent need for individual mobile phone and institutional reporting of at home, hospitalized, and intensive care unit cases of SARS-CoV-2 (COVID-19) infection." *Rev Cardiovasc Med* 2020; 21(1): 1-7.

2. Gautret P, Lagier JC, Parola P, et al. "Hydroxychloroquine and azithromycin as a treatment of COVID-19: results of an open-label non-randomized clinical trial." *Int J Antimicrob Agents* 2020; 56(1): 105949.

3. Risch HA. "Early Outpatient Treatment of Symptomatic, High-Risk COVID-19 Patients That Should Be Ramped Up Immediately as Key to the Pandemic Crisis." *American Journal of Epidemiology* 2020; 189(11): 1218-26.

4. Procter BC, Ross C, Pickard V, Smith E, Hanson C, McCullough PA. "Clinical outcomes after early ambulatory multidrug therapy for high-risk SARS-CoV-2 (COVID-19) infection." *Rev Cardiovasc Med* 2020; 21(4): 611-4.

5. Derwand R, Scholz M, Zelenko V. "COVID-19 outpatients: early risk-stratified treatment with zinc plus low-dose hydroxychloroquine and azithromycin: a retrospective case series study." *International Journal of Antimicrobial Agents* 2020; 56(6): 106214.

6. Ip A, Ahn J, Zhou Y, et al. "Hydroxychloroquine in the treatment of outpatients with mildly symptomatic COVID-19: a multi-center observational study." *BMC Infectious Diseases* 2021; 21(1): 72.

7. Guérin V, Lévy, P., Thomas, J.-L., Lardenois, T., Lacrosse, P., Sarrazin, E., Andreis, N. R.- de, & Wonner, M. "Azithromycin and Hydroxychloroquine Accelerate Recovery of Outpatients with Mild/Moderate COVID-19." *Asian Journal of Medicine and Health* 2020; 18(7): 45-55.

8. Kory P, Meduri GU, Varon J, Iglesias J, Marik PE. "Review of the Emerging Evidence Demonstrating the Efficacy of Ivermectin in the Prophylaxis and Treatment of COVID-19." *Am J Ther* 2021; 28(3): e299-e318.

9. McCullough PA, Oskoui R. "Early multidrug regimens in new potentially fatal medical problems." *Rev Cardiovasc Med* 2020; 21(4): 507-8.

10. McCullough P. "Innovative Early Sequenced Multidrug Therapy for

Sars-Cov-2 (Covid-19) Infection to Reduce Hospitalization and Death." *International Journal of Medical Science and Clinical Invention* 2020; 7(12): 5139-50.

11. Flannery AH, Adkins DA, Cook AM. "Unpeeling the Evidence for the Banana Bag: Evidence-Based Recommendations for the Management of Alcohol-Associated Vitamin and Electrolyte Deficiencies in the ICU." *Crit Care Med* 2016; 44(8): 1545-52.

12. Colbert GB, Venegas-Vera AV, Lerma EV. "Utility of telemedicine in the COVID-19 era." *Rev Cardiovasc Med* 2020; 21(4): 583-7.

13. Savarino A, Boelaert JR, Cassone A, Majori G, Cauda R. "Effects of chloroquine on viral infections: an old drug against today's diseases?" *Lancet Infect Dis* 2003; 3(11): 722-7.

14. Keyaerts E, Vijgen L, Maes P, Neyts J, Van Ranst M. "In vitro inhibition of severe acute respiratory syndrome coronavirus by chloroquine." *Biochem Biophys Res Commun* 2004; 323(1): 264-8.

15. Vincent MJ, Bergeron E, Benjannet S, et al. "Chloroquine is a potent inhibitor of SARS coronavirus infection and spread." *Virology Journal* 2005; 2(1): 69.

16. Rolain JM, Colson P, Raoult D. "Recycling of chloroquine and its hydroxyl analogue to face bacterial, fungal and viral infections in the 21st century." *Int J Antimicrob Agents* 2007; 30(4): 297-308.

17. Sung-sun K. "Physicians work out treatment guidelines for coronavirus." 2.13.2020 2020. http://www.koreabiomed.com/news/articleView.html?idxno=7428.

18. Gao J, Tian Z, Yang X. Breakthrough: "Chloroquine phosphate has shown apparent efficacy in treatment of COVID-19 associated pneumonia in clinical studies." *Biosci Trends* 2020; 14(1): 72-3.

19. Vetter P, Eckerle I, Kaiser L. "Covid-19: a puzzle with many missing pieces." *BMJ* 2020; 368: m627.

20. Pang J, Wang MX, Ang IYH, et al. "Potential Rapid Diagnostics, Vaccine and Therapeutics for 2019 Novel Coronavirus (2019-nCoV): A Systematic Review." *Journal of Clinical Medicine* 2020; 9(3): 623.

21. Colson P, Rolain JM, Lagier JC, Brouqui P, Raoult D. "Chloroquine and

hydroxychloroquine as available weapons to fight COVID-19." *Int J Antimicrob Agents* 2020; 55(4): 105932.

22. Chatterjee P, Anand T, Singh K, et al. Healthcare workers & SARS-CoV-2 infection in India: "A case-control investigation in the time of COVID-19." *Indian Journal of Medical Research* 2020; 151(5): 459-67.

23. Bhattacharya R, Chowdhury S, Nandi A, et al. "Pre-exposure hydroxychloroquine prophylaxis for COVID-19 in healthcare workers: a retrospective cohort." *2020* 2020; 9(1): 8.

24. Berardi F. "The Italian Doctor Flattening the Curve by Treating COVID-19 Patients in Their Homes." TIME. 2020 April 9, 2020.

25. hcqmeta.com. "HCQ for COVID-19: real-time meta analysis of 265 studies." 2021 (accessed July 19, 2021.

26. Consortium WST. "Repurposed Antiviral Drugs for Covid-19—Interim WHO Solidarity Trial Results." *New England Journal of Medicine* 2020; 384(6): 497-511.

27. Group RC. "Effect of Hydroxychloroquine in Hospitalized Patients with Covid-19." *New England Journal of Medicine* 2020; 383(21): 2030-40.

28. Concato J, Shah N, Horwitz RI. "Randomized, Controlled Trials, Observational Studies, and the Hierarchy of Research Designs." *New England Journal of Medicine* 2000; 342(25): 1887-92.

29. Krauss A. "Why all randomised controlled trials produce biased results." *Annals of Medicine* 2018; 50(4): 312-22.

This study remains unpublished in any medical journal for the time being, though the act of publication hardly matters at this stage. One of the things that I discovered while working on this project is that medical science journals strongly prefer research that carries the stamp of approval from an internal review board (IRB). Such boards ostensibly ensure the ethical conduct of science. And for this reason, scientists working on such research only want to put their names on it if that certification is achieved. While that sounds great in theory, the process gets far more complicated than you might imagine.

It turns out that if you're not publishing from an academic institution or public health network with its own IRB, you are at the mercy of the system. Even worse, most well-published scientists, including more than half a dozen I talked with (including my wife), underestimate the bureaucratic labyrinth that entails. This is because their institutions hire specialists in the bureaucracy to handle those details on their behalf. Most never see the sausage getting made. Every single explanation of the system shared with me in emails and phone calls was entirely different from every other one, and one scientist who advised me on some aspects of the paper warned me that moving forward with publication could have legal consequences, though he wasn't really sure what those would be.

If you're thinking that saddling a simple patient case study with a lack of IRB certification for ethical conduct sounds crazy, that's only because you're engaging your common sense.

One well-published research doctor advised us that since Dr. Tyson's and Dr. Fareed's data had already been published and used by the state—that we should be granted an IRB exemption as a quality improvement project (QIP).[44] The study published on some of

---

44 U.S. Department of Health and Human Services. "Quality Improvement Outcome Activities." Retrieved December 7, 2021, from https://www.hhs.gov/ohrp/regulations-and-policy/guidance/faq/quality-improvement-activities/index.html.

Dr. Zelenko's patients was published under a QIP exemption.[45] However, we were turned away after spending two months on our first attempt at obtaining such an exemption, so we haven't even reached the next hurdle of submitting the research to a journal. So much for the rapid review of novel science during an emergency.

After several months of trying to satisfy all parties, we decided to publish the study here in this book. We do also plan to upload it to a preprint server, which is a publicly viewable repository of scientific research that has yet to be accepted for publication in a scientific journal. This may or may not happen ahead of the publication of *Overcoming COVID*. Readers of this book during its first week of publication may be the first to lay their eyes on it.

Publishing delays aside, the reality of the data seems irrelevant to many of the decision-makers, and many others seem hypnotized into ignoring it. Dr. Tyson and Dr. Fareed have given their time for hundreds of interviews, and I posted preliminary results of their work at roundingtheearth.substack.com in May 2021.[46] Other physicians have published their own case series or observational control studies, and nobody at the CDC or FDA cares to aggregate or study the data.

If they did, we would have had a dashboard following the evolution of progress of all forms of frontline medical care and their results from the start of the pandemic. Such a dashboard would have looked less scary than the Johns Hopkins dashboard showing big red blots dotting

---

45 Derwand, Roland et al. "COVID-19 outpatients: early risk-stratified treatment with zinc plus low-dose hydroxychloroquine and azithromycin: a retrospective case series study." *International journal of antimicrobial agents* vol. 56,6 (2020): 106214. doi:10.1016/j.ijantimicag.2020.106214.

46 Crawford, M. (May 13, 2021). "Why The Early Treatment Data is Better Than Anyone Imagines: Dr. Brian Tyson's Data." Retrieved December 7, 2021, from https://roundingtheearth.substack.com/p/the-chloroquine-wars-part-xx.

the globe,[47] and would have encouraged those infected with SARS-CoV-2 to seek and prepare medical treatment early, which is the only option that ever made sense.

Since the compilation of the data that went into our study, Dr. Tyson and Dr. Fareed have treated many more patients, and with similar results. If we broke the numbers down into Protocol 1 (prior to ivermectin's addition), Protocol 2 (from ivermectin's addition to the end of our study), and Protocol 3 (since the end of our study inclusion period), we would have three highly similar protocols with three highly similar outcomes: zero deaths and one to two hospitalizations for each of three groups. These groups are of 1,585 to well over 2,000 COVID-19 patients, all treated starting in the early stages of COVID-19 symptoms, or even earlier for high-risk presymptomatic patients.

How is all this evidence of the efficacy of the early treatment paradigm not convincing to everyone? Why weren't 2,000 patients with no deaths enough? What about 4,000? What about when Dr. Tyson and Dr. Fareed passed 6,000 and kept tallying a perfect record? When around 30 out of every 1,000 residents of Imperial County who became ill from COVID-19, not treated by AVUC died, how many AVUC patients need to recover without a death before an open mind thinks, "Maybe there's something to this?"

I grew up watching the Los Angeles Lakers dominate professional basketball. I recall believing that Irving "Magic" Johnson, a guy who could play any position on the court and smile doing it, was the world's best basketball player. For a few years, maybe he was. But I continued

---

47 Johns Hopkins University. Coronavirus Resource Center. Retrieved December 7, 2021 from https://coronavirus.jhu.edu/map.html.

to believe that was still the case even after Michael Jordan continuously hovered forty-eight inches off the ground while dominating the Lakers to earn his first NBA championship ring. At some point, somewhere between Jordan's first championship ring and his sixth (Second? Third?), I accepted reality over Magic.

Why?

Repetition and *consistency* are powerfully convincing, and Jordan won big game after big game, and championship after championship, even on nights when he was sick with just the flu. If, like me, you found yourself rooting for the teams that rivaled his Chicago Bulls, you had to accept the reality of his dominance—even when it felt maddening to behold.

Almost everyone else accepted Jordan's basketball superiority, too. It was simply a matter of how many games that reality took to sink in. *Repetition* and *consistency*. For those watching Jordan play every night, it probably didn't take long. For those of us usually watching other teams, then comparing box scores and statistical compilations, we had to work through the ways in which we weighed the results. But the ultimate results in basketball are wins and championships, and Jordan's Bulls dominated those statistics with *repetition* and *consistency*. In a room of a hundred basketball fans, you could always find that guy still arguing hopelessly for Magic or Charles Barkley or Kareen Olajuwon, depending on the season, but most everyone else came around: Jordan was the greatest of the era, if not of all time.

And nobody needed an RCT to tell them Jordan was the court king of the 1990s. If you didn't get it after so much *repetition* and *consistency*, we all rolled our eyes and took a mental note of the nature of your biases.

And if you're thinking that such a judgment over the efficacy of athletes in winning contests for unusually tall people is fundamentally different from the judgments made by scientists about drug efficacy in treating rapidly spreading viruses, you are mistaken. Evaluation of statistical results has few hard and fast rules, and relating those results to reality is its own academic task that can spark debate. What a good professional statistician or scientist does is the same as what any curious mind does: go deep asking questions about the nature of results. It's a lot like what sports fans do, but with more training— sometimes for the better, and apparently sometimes for the worse.

Given that there is no large-scale early treatment RCT data, how much data do you need to see to decide that a drug probably works? How much *repetition* and *consistency* do you need before you change your mind?

When I ask this question, as I often have, I don't think I've heard a straight answer. That troubles me. I can understand taking some time to think about it, but dodging the question suggests a motivation to dodge the issue. A straight answer would require declaring a *threshold—* a barrier for acceptance that *could* be surpassed. If somebody gives an answer: 1,000 or 5,000 or 20,000 or 100,000, they commit to acceptance of the result when the data arrives. That's a scary proposition for those who—for whatever reason—are *invested* in suppressing an answer. For a scientist or statistician with an open mind, it's just a number, whether or not it's the perfectly economical number.

But the Gods of Public Health tell us from their perch that only randomized control trials (RCTs) can give us an acceptable answer, so *there is no number.* Were there a nation that treated a billion patients without a death, it would not matter to them. They would find some reason (a "confounder") and declare that without an RCT, we'll never know whether it was the medication that prevented so many deaths, or whether it was perhaps the fact that those billion people work together better in any and all circumstances. While most approved medications never underwent an RCT, regulatory officials now declare there is no "proof" without one, but that's not how statistics works, and "proof" has no meaning in the context of either science or statistics.

For those not steeped in an understanding of the branches of philosophy we call logic, mathematics, and science, there is only *proof* in the context of logical systems, used often in mathematics.[48] To the extent that we write proofs over the course of statistical analysis of scientific evidence, these are generally mundane statements about numerical limits (such as a minimum or maximum values of calculations), but never in the context of, "We know as *truth* the implication of these experimental results. We *proved* it." The incorrect and manipulative use of such fundamental terminology is a hallmark of some public health bureaucrats such as Dr. Anthony Fauci.

Honest statisticians respect *repetition* and *consistency* and work to quantify its presence or absence as best as possible within the context of more and less perfect circumstances.

Aside from the con men at the tops of various medical hierarchies, there are a lot of serious players falling into line with pronouncements of failure in the use of hydroxychloroquine to prevent or treat COVID-19. In July, I exchanged emails with Stanford Professor John Ioannidis. Upon hearing about the amazing results at AVUC, he responded, "Confidentially: 99.74% is roughly the survival of sixty-year-olds when they are infected with COVID-19 in the absence of any treatment. So, I am not much convinced by Fareed and Tyson . . ."

---

48   *Stanford Encycloedia of Philosophy.* (August 13, 2018). "Proof Theory." Retrieved December 7, 2021 from https://plato.stanford.edu/entries/proof-theory/.

Why was he comparing the **survival rate** of *one demographic slice* with the **relative risk reduction of hospitalization** between two *more general cohorts*?

I'm still scratching my head over how to interpret his nonsequitur, but I responded, "For Tyson and Fareed, the 99.74% was hospitalization reduction relative to county averages. Out of 3,962 patients, two were hospitalized and zero died," thinking that Professor Ioannidis read the discussion too quickly to understand what he was reading (I am sure he is a busy man—I have misread my own share of emails during the pandemonium, and I try to be generous on that level).

His reply baffled me: "For their demographics, one would expect zero-to-three deaths without treatment and between zero and ten hospitalizations," dismissing the results as not meaningful without (as he put it) "rigorous RCTs."

Where were these calculations coming from? I never sent him the demographics data. He made this statement without knowing the age or health profiles of the patients. I've had a few thousand conversations with professional statisticians and quantitative analysts, but not many that involved what appears to be the conjuring of numerical ranges out of thin air, entirely unsupported by data, models, or methodology. This man is supposed to be one of the world's leading applied statisticians in epidemiology and medicine, teaching on these disciplines at one of the world's premier universities.

I replied, "John, I performed a mapping from their patient pool to the county's and came up with around sixty lives saved for that pool of patients," referring to the 3,962 patients in Protocols 1 or 2, which does not take into account lives saved among those treated already at a moderate or severe stage of COVID-19, or the other patients treated by Dr. Fareed, some of whom were in the very high-risk patient pool that includes nursing home patients. While personal confidence in such an estimate is wide, a suggestion like his that the true mortality rate would be 95% to 100% lower than that needs explaining—particularly in a county where over 3% of COVID-19 cases resulted in death.

Professor Ioannidis responded again, saying that he didn't think that *any* lives were saved at AVUC, "But in the absence of a real solid control, any interpretation is open." He also tossed in a suggestion that I was confusing two metrics of mortality (infection fatality rate and case fatality rate), though without asking any questions to find out how I was using terminology, much less reviewing any data to come to that conclusion.

In my follow-up, I let him know that the comparison was apples-to-apples (case fatality rates), and that I had confirmed the cases with the county epidemiologist (which I took the step to do both by phone and then also in email to secure documentation). His suggestion, without knowing the details, of such a basic error struck me as a subtle kind of intellectual bullying. Science doesn't begin with a conclusion, then work its way backward, rearranging or attacking data that doesn't fit the hypothesis. Historically speaking, whether Galileo Galilee, Roger Bacon, Ibn al-Haytham, or somebody else was the first to employ it, that sort of reasoning is precisely what the scientific method was invented to combat.

I remained polite, but upped the ante. These cases were no different in definition than the 21,000 or so other cases in the county that took over 600 lives through March 2021, and I wanted him to look at the data and hoped to engage in a more reasonable discussion from there. Sometimes stubborn people give in and work well after prying the door open, right? I also wanted to let him know that I was ready to defend the conclusion I believed in after putting in the effort, "Yes, we are talking about in the ballpark of several scores lives saved. As I've said, I am happy to confirm with Tyson's permission to forward data if you would like to have a look. I am sure he will not mind."

Tired of what I felt was a game with an implied starting point of, "we hoped hydroxychloroquine worked, but it failed," I pointed out, "nearly all the evidence against HCQ came from late-stage studies. If we are interested in a drug's efficacy, it only makes sense that we examine its optimal use protocol. How many studies suggest a failure for early treatment?"

Part of what I was getting at was the absurdity of the WHO trials that tested the worst imaginable protocols for hydroxychloroquine.[49] Even while dozens of nations used highly similar protocols, and doctors from some of those nations spoke out in objection to the WHO protocols, the WHO moved forward with protocols entirely dissimilar to those used anywhere else. They refused to respect the value of *repetition* and *consistency*.

Supposedly, these large RCTs demonstrated that hydroxychloroquine was ineffective in the treatment of COVID-19. But the study parameters were all wrong, and in all possible ways. Contradicting the WHO's own review of pharmacokinetic research that suggested the physicians around the world using mostly 2.4g to 4g of hydroxychloroquine was optimal, they chose doses 2.5 to more than 4 times that high![50]

Then they administered these doses without zinc, the conjunctive element of the most effective hydroxychloroquine therapies, or any other of the companion vitamins or macrolides used by Dr. Tyson,

49 Crawford, M. (June 13, 2021). "How to Rig Research: The WHO Edition." Retrieved December 7, 2021, from https://roundingtheearth.substack.com/p/how-to-rig-research-the-who-edition.
50 Crawford, M. (June 13, 2021). "How to Rig Research: The WHO Edition." Retrieved December 7, 2021, from https://roundingtheearth.substack.com/p/how-to-rig-research-the-who-edition.

Dr. Fareed, or the many other physicians seeing excellent outcomes. Further, they only treated patients with hydroxychloroquine many days after patients were sick, which is after most viral replication has subsided and the resulting disease state mechanism no longer depends on the presence of a live virus. In fact, most of the patients treated this way were already on supplemental oxygen.[51] Who could possibly defend such a study as appropriate, much less conclude that it disproves the efficacy of more reasonable protocols?

WHO indeed.

Hydroxychloroquine Protocol Comparison

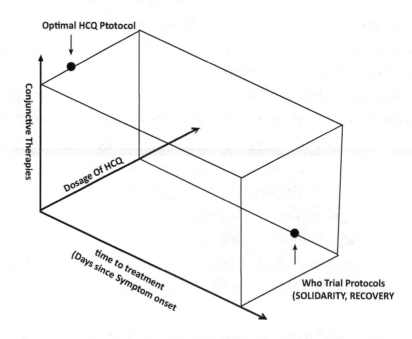

51 Crawford, M. (June 13, 2021). "How to Rig Research: The WHO Edition." Retrieved December 7, 2021, from https://roundingtheearth.substack.com/p/how-to-rig-research-the-who-edition.

How does anyone confuse these medical treatment protocols as the same? Or even remotely similar?

No reply ever followed from Professor Ioannidis.

Hydroxychloroquine Early Treatment and Pre-exposure Prophylaxis Studies (Studies on immunocompromised patients excluded)

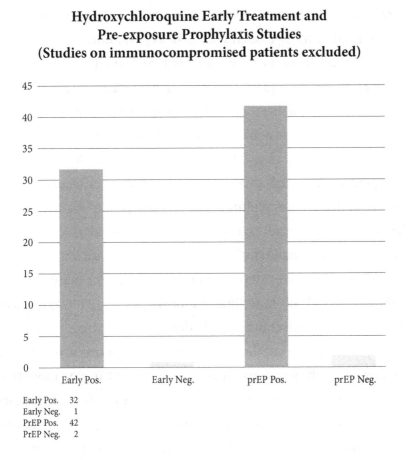

Early Pos.	32
Early Neg.	1
PrEP Pos.	42
PrEP Neg.	2

Above is a summary of effects reported from the early treatment research on hydroxychloroquine as of December 8, 2021, though all or nearly all of these studies were known at the time I tried to engage with Professor Ioannidis. In all, there were over thirty early treatment studies on hydroxychloroquine's effects on COVID-19 patients published or in preprint. Among them, we see great *repetition* and *consistency*.

In just one of the studies, the control arm outperformed the treatment arm. In that small study on eighty-four total patients,[52] there was *one hospitalization*, which occurred in the treatment arm. Within such a small and healthy study pool of those eighty-four patients, we might check other measured outcomes to better understand the results. It turns out that those treated with hydroxychloroquine in the study saw faster clearance of the virus measured from zero to three to six and to nine days from the start of treatment. It would be interesting to find out if the one hospitalized patient had some unexamined condition like the auto-interferon antibody disorder that has been reported to be associated with as much as 20% of all COVID-19 deaths.[53]

Regardless, one such small study is not at all inconsistent with the hypothesis that hydroxychloroquine is a key part of a cocktail that, when used early or prior to disease protection, results in substantial benefits. Out of so many studies, unless all of them are large (which is not the case) or include sufficient numbers of high-risk individuals, we would certainly expect to see one or more negative outcomes, even for highly effective medications, simply due to chance alone.

Why? Because even Michael Jordan lost games. If you flip a fair coin long enough, you'll eventually see streaks of five or more tails. Rare events happen, and these kinds of events are not even all that rare.

At the time of the writing of this book, there are eleven studies out of India that tested the use of hydroxychloroquine as a pre-exposure

---

52   Rodrigues, Cristhieni et al. "Hydroxychloroquine plus azithromycin early treatment of mild COVID-19 in an outpatient setting: a randomized, double-blinded, placebo-controlled clinical trial evaluating viral clearance." *International journal of antimicrobial agents* vol. 58,5 (2021): 106428. doi:10.1016/j.ijantimicag.2021.106428

53   Bastard, Paul et al. "Autoantibodies neutralizing type I IFNs are present in ~4% of uninfected individuals over 70 years old and account for ~20% of COVID-19 deaths." *Science immunology* vol. 6,62 (2021): eabl4340. doi:10.1126/sciimmunol.abl4340.

prophylaxis. In every single one of them, those who received hydroxychloroquine suffered a lower incidence of COVID-19 than those who received a placebo.[54] A total of six of those studies tested dose dependency, meaning they also compared the results of those who took hydroxychloroquine for at least six weeks straight. In each of those studies, those taking the drug for at least six weeks suffered a lower incident of COVID-19 than those who took the drug for less time or not at all. These trials stand out as a dramatic demonstration of *repetition* and *consistency*.

I've thought about why Professor Ioannidis never replied to my last email in our exchange. The conversation was energetic, but polite. This is often where science gets really good—with the tension of two or more curious parties, believing two versions of a story, but willing to dive in, splash around, and make noise while trying to sort it all out. Except that he never splashed around. Instead of getting his feet wet with the data collected at the front lines of medicine, he just disappeared from the conversation.

Personally, I think that statistics can never be worth more than the value of the data source, so I tend to take every invitation to get closer to the source, so long as it's economical to do so. In this case, Professor Ioannidis would have received the data I'd already taken the pains to clean and verify with the county. For free. He could have connected with Dr. Tyson and Dr. Fareed with little effort, but he chose not to.

Since that exchange, I've been on at least one additional email exchange with Professor Ioannidis. He said that the vaccines had

---

54 Stricker, Raphael B, and Melissa C Fesler. "Hydroxychloroquine Pre-Exposure Prophylaxis for COVID-19 in Healthcare Workers from India: A Meta-Analysis." *Journal of infection and public health* vol. 14,9 (2021): 1161-1163. doi:10.1016/j.jiph.2021.08.001.

saved lives, which I suppose means that he is willing to take the trial reports directly from vaccine manufacturers (with scores of criminal convictions, or else zero experience bringing products to market) as RCTs at face value, even though their reports read neither as random nor blinded. Professor Ioannidis may be most famous for opening broad dialogue in the scientific community over the replication crisis of published scientific results that often cannot be reproduced in attempts by other researchers.[55] Here it seems that we have well-replicated results of early ambulatory medical treatment (and also prophylaxis), and highly inconsistent indicators of vaccine efficacy in the published literature. Perhaps as of the pandemic, the new crisis in science is that of replicability of *standards of evidence.*

Professor Ioannidis may be the most credentialed, but he is far from the only academic or physician I've encountered whose dismissal of overwhelmingly positive early treatment data baffled me. When looking back at the many conversations I've had, one thing I notice about those early treatment denialists is a strange and deliberate lack of contact with any of the physicians making use of hydroxychloroquine, ivermectin, quercetin, or other medications at the first sign of illness.

What kind of sense does it make to form deeply held convictions about a medical or scientific topic entirely at a distance? Have we forgotten how millions of sailors died of scurvy because physicians sitting in privileged halls of elite societies declared that vitamin C (or specifically the fruits that contained it) was not the proven variable while ship captains and the on-site doctors who traveled with them

---

55 Ioannidis, John P A. "Why most published research findings are false." *PLoS medicine* vol. 2, 8 (2005): e124. doi:10.1371/journal.pmed.0020124.

argued *for centuries* that they saw the evidence of the connection with their own eyes?[56] Wasn't that our cautionary tale about trusting a medical establishment tied to corporate profits (based on available cargo space that such fruits would have taken up) over the practice of empiric medicine?

Perhaps we need to take a look back to the early days of the pandemic, and a bit further back than that, to best understand the resistance to early treatment medications in the present and historically unique context. On March 19, 2020, President Donald Trump took the podium at a press conference, speaking optimistically about two drugs for which the FDA gave emergency approval: hydroxychloroquine and remdesivir.[57]

"So you have remdesivir and you have hydroxychloroquine. So those are two that are out now, essentially approved for prescribed use. And I think it's going to be very exciting. I think it could be a game-changer, and maybe not and maybe not, but I think it could be, based on what I see, it could be a game-changer. Very powerful. They're very powerful."

Trump also spoke about hydroxychloroquine's long track record and excellent safety profile. Somehow, within the span of a few hours, a large portion of the media determined with great confidence that hydroxychloroquine, a drug consumed by humans worldwide to the

---

56 Crawford, M. (May 11, 2021). "Historical Failures of Public Health Authorities." Retrieved December 7, 2021, from https://roundingtheearth.substack.com/p/the-chloroquine-wars-part-xix.

57 Rev Transcript Library. (March 19, 2020). "Donald Trump Coronavirus Task Force Briefing Transcript March 19: Trump Takes Shots at the Media." Retrieved December 7, 2021, from https://www.rev.com/blog/transcripts/donald-trump-coronavirus-task-force-briefing-transcript-march-19-trump-takes-shots-at-the-media.

tune of many tens of billions of doses over the past several decades, was mockworthy, dangerous snake oil.[58]

I've never had a great deal of confidence in the press, and even less in most of the so-called "science media," but the suddenness of the snake oil proclamation stunned me. Was a large portion of the media somehow privy to research that the public was not? Is that why there was no buzz at all about doctors using hydroxychloroquine? Wouldn't *that* have been its own story?! And if medical doctors and associated academics were not speaking out *en masse* in shock of the media's declaration of danger and inefficacy of a relatively safe drug, what was stopping them? Was there some central machinery distributed incentives or marching orders to squelch the story of hydroxychloroquine's efficacy? The signs of organized behind-the-scenes communication were there, but let's take a closer look at the details before we jump to any conclusions.

As I began my own investigation into what was going on, I found out that many physicians had already been prescribing it to patients prior to Trump's chat with the press. They all felt positive about it, and none reported seeing harsh side effects with patients, heart-related or otherwise. Why was there no buzz about this in the press? Maybe there was, and I just missed it?

On March 23, 2020, Christopher Rowland published an article in the Washington Post under a headline that complained about a run on supplies of hydroxychloroquine that could harm chronic users, such as sufferers of lupus and rheumatoid arthritis.[59] This "run"

---

58 Crawford, M. (April 9, 2021). "The Chloroquine Wars Part XII: Manufactured Fear During Hydroxychloroquine's Trump Moment." Retrieved December 7, 2021, from https://roundingtheearth.substack.com/p/the-chloroquine-wars-part-xii.

59 Rowland, C. (March 23, 2020). "As Trump touts an unproven coronavirus treatment, supplies evaporate for patients

proved to be highly localized to a small handful of pharmacies, and extremely short-lived. There has never been evidence that anyone who needed the drug for their chronic condition failed to obtain it, and hydroxychloroquine remains stable in the bloodstream for days to weeks, meaning that missing a day or two of medication is not generally problematic. However, buried in the article was this revealing fact:

"Data gathered in the first 17 days of March by Premier Inc., a large group purchasing organization for 4,000 U.S. hospitals, showed a 300 percent week-over-week increase in orders of chloroquine and a 70 percent week-over-week boost in orders of hydroxychloroquine."

In other words, many hospitals (meaning likely essentially all of them) *already knew* that chloroquine and hydroxychloroquine were considered by coronavirus researchers to be the best shots at treating COVID-19 before Trump's press conference introduced the medications to the larger public consciousness. Either *the collective sum of all major Western media outlets* failed to discover that fact before Trump spoke, or there was organized suppression of the information.

But to the article's headline point, hydroxychloroquine manufacturers had already offered to donate well over 100 million doses of hydroxychloroquine to fight COVID-19,[60] and Trump had created a national stockpile to ensure supply of the drug immediately after his

who need those drugs." *Washington Post*. Retrieved December 7, 2021, from https://www.washingtonpost.com/business/2020/03/20/hospitals-doctors-are-wiping-out-supplies-an-unproven-coronavirus-treatment/.

60 Crawford, M. (April 9, 2021). "The Chloroquine Wars Part XII: Manufactured Fear During Hydroxychloroquine's Trump Moment". Retrieved December 7, 2021, from https://roundingtheearth.substack.com/p/the-chloroquine-wars-part-xii.

press conference.[61] That didn't keep some corners of the media from pushing the supply scare story for months afterward.

As my conversations expanded to include doctors on multiple continents, the story remained largely the same: many doctors in Asia and Europe were already using hydroxychloroquine to treat patients. So, why then, when I used Google or other search engines to find out more about hydroxychloroquine usage up to March 19, 2020, was I finding almost no discussion at all about it? (I encourage readers to perform their own searches in date ranges up to March 18, 2020.)

To be sure, I did get a scarce few relevant hits in my searches:

- On February 6, in an article in the niche publication *ASBMB Today* (American Society for Biochemistry and Molecular Biology), science writer John Arnst pointed out that scientists at the Wuhan Institute of Virology were already claiming the evidence of the efficacy of chloroquine.[62]
- On February 13, the English-language news outlet *China Daily* published an article identifying hydroxychloroquine as a potential treatment for SARS-CoV-2 infection.[63]
- On February 20, Nigerian journalist Adekanye Modupeoluwa referenced the enthusiasm of a Nigerian physician over chloroquine in a *Guardian Nigeria* article.[64]

61 AAP. (April 9, 2020). "Nearly 30 million Hydroxychloroquine pills in national stockpile: Trump." *News.com*. Retrieved December 7, 2021, from https://www.news.com.au/world/nearly-30-million-hydroxychloroquine-pills-in-national-stockpile-trump/video/9066cada9131da69fa0b47d292ff5d05.

62 Arnst, J. (February 6, 2020). "Could an old malaria drug help fight the new coronavirus?" *ASBMBToday*. https://www.asbmb.org/asbmb-today/science/020620/could-an-old-malaria-drug-help-fight-the-new-coron.

63 Yi, X. (February 13, 2020). "Malaria drug identified as potential treatment for novel coronavirus." *ChinaDaily.com.cn*. Retrieved December 7, 2021, from https://www.chinadaily.com.cn/a/202002/13/WS5e45222ca310128217277606.ht ml?fbclid=IwAR2vDjTAizgg7NaFgnJxzt8NU-VGi1f7ElfUOZcnrzsBZxocwH8beLCKQDY.

64 Adekanye, M. (February 20, 2020). "NIGERIANS REACT TO USE OF CHLOROQUINE FOR FIGHTING CORONAVIRUS." *The*

- The parent outlet, *The Guardian*, seems not to have followed up on the story itself.

- On February 25 and 26, a couple of interviews by the French research physician and professor, Dr. Didier Raoult—speaking of the hope of hydroxychloroquine in ending the pandemic—were uploaded and available.[65, 66] American media never bothered to translate or report on them.

- On February 26, the United Kingdom added chloroquine to the list of medicines illegal to export, perhaps to ensure domestic supply.[67] but that failed to draw the attention of any of the razor-sharp reporters covering the pandemic.

- On March 10, the popular medical education producer MedCram featured a video expressing "cautious optimism" over COVID-19 treatment with chloroquine and zinc.[68]

- On March 11, the University of Oxford registered the COPCOV trial to study the potential for chloroquine and hydroxychloroquine to prevent COVID-19.[69]

- On March 17, the University of Minnesota posted a press release announcing an RCT testing hydroxychloroquine as a post-exposure

Guardian (Nigeria). Retrieved December 7, 2021, from https://guardian.ng/life/nigerians-react-to-use-of-chloroquine-for-fighting-coronavirus/.

65 https://youtu.be/8L6ehRif-v8

66 https://www.20minutes.fr/sante/2727411-20200226-coronavirus-faute-medicale-donner-chloroquine-contre-virus-chinois-selon-professeur-didier-raoult.

67 GlobalData Healthcare. (March 13, 2020). "UK bans parallel export and hoarding of three Covid-19 drugs." *Pharmaceutical Technology*. Retrieved December 7, 2021, from https://www.pharmaceutical-technology.com/comment/parallel-export-covid-19/.

68 MedCram – Medical Lectures Explained CLEARLY. (March 10, 2020). "Coronavirus Epidemic Update 34: US Cases Surge, Chloroquine & Zinc Treatment Combo, Italy Lockdown." Retrieved December 7, 2021, from https://youtu.be/U7F1cnWup9M.

69 ClinicalTrials.gov. (March 11, 2020). "Chloroquine/ Hydroxychloroquine Prevention of Coronavirus Disease (COVID-19) in the Healthcare Setting (COPCOV)." Retrieved December 7, 2021, from https://clinicaltrials.gov/ct2/show/NCT04303507.

prophylactic to prevent COVID-19.[70] Somehow that didn't catch anyone's eye in the media for at least a few days.

- There was a single discussion about these drugs in a Reddit post that I found from late February.[71]

Otherwise, there was essentially no *visible* discussion of these potential antivirals in the Western media, including the medical media, in my internet searches.[72] Certainly, nothing that was easily obtainable and digestible by the public.

Now, let us be clear that what we are talking about are potentially repurposed drugs. That is to say that we are investigating the hypothesis that medicines that were successful in the prevention and treatment of other ailments, like the malaria caused by parasites, also work against the virus we call SARS-CoV-2. Most attempts at repurposing drugs fail, but for economic reasons, we tend to look for reapplications of already known medicines rather than researching new ones—particularly those that have a proven safety record and are inexpensive. Chloroquine and hydroxychloroquine are among the least expensive drugs to produce, ranging from a fraction of a dollar to a little over a dollar per dose to manufacture.

Should we *expect* hydroxychloroquine to fail in this case?

In a November 2020 article in *The Journal of the American Academy of Psychiatry and the Law*, researchers noted one medical prescription

---

70   Glynn, K. (March 17, 2020). "COVID-19 Clinical Trial Launches at University of Minnesota." *University of Minnesota.* Retrieved December 7, 2021, from https://med.umn.edu/news-events/covid-19-clinical-trial-launches-university-minnesota.

71   WallachianVoivode. (February 26, 2020). "Hydroxychloroquine (Plaquenil) thread." *Reddit.* Retrieved December 7, 2021, from https://www.reddit.com/r/COVID19/comments/f9sozs/hydroxychloroquine_plaquenil_thread/.

72   Crawford, M. (March 3, 2021). "The Curious Calm Before the Storm." Retrieved December 7, 2021, from https://roundingtheearth.substack.com/p/the-chloroquine-wars-part-ii.

review that found 21% of prescriptions for medications commonly used in general office-based practice are off-label.[73] These are repurposed drugs for conditions other than the ones for which they were initially approved. I have seen estimates of off-label prescriptions higher than 50%. Regardless of the exact proportion, it is clear that repurposed drugs are often found to work, and for a wide variety of conditions.

As it turns out, hydroxychloroquine is about the most repurposed drug in the history of medicine, used to treat parasites, bacterial infections, a host of over a dozen auto-immune disorders, and has shown broad antiviral properties in testing.[74] Medical researchers are even exploring its use as a unique cancer medication due to its unusual combination of attributes.[75] But none of that matters if hydroxychloroquine cannot inhibit SARS-CoV-2 or quell the symptoms of COVID-19, so why should we think it has any more potential than any of the thousands of other potentially repurposed drugs?

As I dug into the literature, I found a substantial body of research detailing both practical and mechanistic reasons to believe that hydroxychloroquine very well could treat viruses, and SARS-like coronaviruses in particular! There are references in medical literature to hydroxychloroquine's active precursor, quinine, being used successfully to treat both the Russian flu and the Spanish flu.[76, 77]

73 Shariful A. Syed, Brigham A. Dixson, Eduardo Constantino, Judith Regan. "The Law and Practice of Off-Label Prescribing and Physician Promotion". Journal of the American Academy of Psychiatry and the Law Online Nov 2020, JAAPL.200049-20; DOI: 10.29158/JAAPL.200049-20.

74 Crawford, M. (March 2, 2021). "Drugs of the Cinchona Tree." Retrieved December 7, 2021, from https://roundingtheearth.substack.com/p/the-chloroquine-wars-part-i.

75 Cook, Katherine L et al. "Hydroxychloroquine inhibits autophagy to potentiate antiestrogen responsiveness in ER+ breast cancer." *Clinical cancer research : an official journal of the American Association for Cancer Research* vol. 20,12 (2014): 3222-32. doi:10.1158/1078-0432.CCR-13-3227.

76 https://wellcomecollection.org/works/zkse3qja/

77 https://c19study.com/burrows.html

More specifically, there are numerous papers published in the years following the first SARS coronavirus epidemic that indicate powerfully successful use of chloroquine or hydroxychloroquine as SARS coronavirus inhibitors.[78, 79, 80] Other research demonstrated zinc's success in blocking coronavirus replication,[81] indicating the potential for all agents that help zinc get into cells, such as chloroquine and hydroxychloroquine,[82, 83] to help prevent infection and spread of coronaviruses.

While obviously not specific to SARS-CoV-2, which would not be known to the scientific community for years to come, the researchers in the papers specific to coronaviruses often went to lengths to suggest that chloroquine and hydroxychloroquine should be *the first two drugs off the shelf* to be tested for efficacy during the next deadly coronavirus outbreak. Add to that additional rationale letters written by scientists and physicians in both China (where SARS-CoV-2 was first publicly identified) and the West unanimously recommended giving chloroquine and hydroxychloroquine a try in treating COVID-19, and we have very good reason to view the potential of these two drugs

78 Savarino, Andrea et al. "Effects of chloroquine on viral infections: an old drug against today's diseases?" *The Lancet. Infectious diseases* vol. 3,11 (2003): 722-7. doi:10.1016/s1473-3099(03)00806-5.

79 Keyaerts, Els et al. "In vitro inhibition of severe acute respiratory syndrome coronavirus by chloroquine." *Biochemical and biophysical research communications* vol. 323,1 (2004): 264-8. doi:10.1016/j.bbrc.2004.08.085.

80 Vincent, Martin J et al. "Chloroquine is a potent inhibitor of SARS coronavirus infection and spread." *Virology journal* vol. 2 69. 22 Aug. 2005, doi:10.1186/1743-422X-2-69.

81 te Velthuis, Aartjan J W et al. "Zn(2+) inhibits coronavirus and arterivirus RNA polymerase activity in vitro and zinc ionophores block the replication of these viruses in cell culture." *PLoS pathogens* vol. 6,11 e1001176. 4 Nov. 2010, doi:10.1371/journal.ppat.1001176.

82 Xue, Jing et al. "Chloroquine is a zinc ionophore." *PLoS one* vol. 9,10 e109180. 1 Oct. 2014, doi:10.1371/journal. pone.0109180.

83 Dabbagh-Bazarbachi, Husam et al. "Zinc ionophore activity of quercetin and epigallocatechin-gallate: from Hepa 1-6 cells to a liposome model." *Journal of agricultural and food chemistry* vol. 62,32 (2014): 8085-93. doi:10.1021/jf5014633.

as fundamentally different from that of a randomly selected drug to repurpose.[84]

There was one single repurposed drug rationale paper published that made no mention of either chloroquine or hydroxychloroquine. That was the one published on January 23, 2020, in the Journal of American Medicine, written by Dr. Catharine Paules, Dr. Hilary Marston, and Dr. Anthony Fauci.[85] A letter to the editor received by the journal *Cell Research* just two days later documents positive *in vitro* experiments at the Wuhan Institute of Virology involving these drugs.[86] From that letter:

"Our time-of-addition assay demonstrated that chloroquine functioned at both entry, and at post-entry stages of the 2019-nCoV infection in Vero E6 cells . . ."

The initially used name for SARS-CoV-2 was 2019-nCoV. Was Dr. Fauci, the director of the NIAID, truly unaware of that report by that time? Was what was going on in *China*, the epicenter of the outbreak, outside of his attention span? Or did he have some reason, unknown to the entire field of infectious disease researchers, to believe that neither chloroquine nor hydroxychloroquine would demonstrate efficacy in preventing or treating SARS-CoV-2 infection in humans? Maybe he was too busy wondering what to do with emails from researchers concerned that SARS-CoV-2 looked manmade.[87]

---

84 Crawford, M. (March 3, 2021). "The Curious Calm Before the Storm." Retrieved December 7, 2021, from https://roundingtheearth.substack.com/p/the-chloroquine-wars-part-ii.

85 https://jamanetwork.com/journals/jama/fullarticle/2759815?resultClick=1

86 Wang, Manli et al. "Remdesivir and chloroquine effectively inhibit the recently emerged novel coronavirus (2019-nCoV) in vitro." *Cell research* vol. 30,3 (2020): 269-271. doi:10.1038/s41422-020-0282-0.

87 Crawford, M. (June 7, 2021). "The Fauci Emails: Truth Finally Uncovered, or a Bishop Sacrifice?" Retrieved December 7, 2021, from https://roundingtheearth.substack.com/p/the-fauci-emails-truth-finally-uncovered.

If Dr. Fauci did have some reason to exclude hydroxychloroquine from the list of repurposed drugs with potential, he has never made that clear. He later behaved as if the proposition of hydroxychloroquine efficacy was almost at random, and like he was taking a wait-and-see approach. The NIH eventually launched a trial on May 14, 2020,[88] purportedly to study whether hydroxychloroquine and azithromycin prevented hospitalization or death when used early, so perhaps Dr. Fauci's exclusion of hydroxychloroquine from his preferred list was merely ignorant oversight? That NIH trial, which was to include 2,000 participants, was halted after just five weeks. In a bulletin published by the NIH, they claimed inadequate trial enrollment,[89] but they had not even waited for the summer COVID-19 wave, which basically began the week in June that the trial was halted.

So, there were tens of thousands of Americans willing to line up for experimental gene therapy trials, but the NIH couldn't locate 2,000 infected Americans willing to test the efficacy of a repurposed drug with a well-known safety profile when the alternative was generally to just wait and get sick enough to be hospitalized and maybe placed on a ventilator? The totality of these stories pushes me beyond mere skepticism. It all strikes me as bat-CoV insane.

Now, let's rewind for a moment. Despite the lack of attention given to the topic by U.S. public health authorities or the mainstream media, there *was* summary information about the use of hydroxychloroquine

---

88 NIAID. (March 14, 2020). "NIH Begins Clinical Trial of Hydroxychloroquine and Azithromycin to Treat COVID-19." Retrieved December 7, 2021, from https://www.niaid.nih.gov/news-events/nih-begins-clinical-trial-hydroxychloroquine-and-azithromycin-treat-covid-19.

89 NIAID. (June 20, 2020). "BULLETIN—NIH Clinical Trial Evaluating Hydroxychloroquine and Azithromycin for COVID-19 Closes Early." Retrieved December 7, 2021, from https://www.niaid.nih.gov/news-events/bulletin-nih-clinical-trial-evaluating-hydroxychloroquine-and-azithromycin-covid-19.

in the prevention and treatment of COVID-19 available on the internet for the American audience prior to Trump's press conference introducing the topic. On March 13, 2020, Dr. James Todaro and his friend Gregory Rigano published an educational fifteen-page document entitled, "An Effective Treatment for Coronavirus (COVID-19)" directly on the internet in the form of a Google document.[90] The document covered a summary of the research and rationales already known at the time, and some notes about treatment guidelines for the use of chloroquine and hydroxychloroquine in China and South Korea where they were already in for several weeks. Three days later, Elon Musk tweeted out Dr. Todaro's and Rigano's paper to his tens of millions of followers.[91]

On March 18, 2020, it seems that Google decided to censor that document one day prior to Trump's first public mention of hydroxychloroquine.[92] As a result, the millions of Americans for whom "hydroxychloroquine" was a complicated and unfamiliar word, found little to nothing about its growing international use, or the historical research suggesting it as the first best option to try.

Can there be any doubt that the deafening media silence about the potential for chloroquine and hydroxychloroquine was coordinated? Does it seem likely that the hundreds of articles proclaiming its danger or premature announcing its failure were meant to fill that void,

90 Todary, J., Rigano, G., (March 13, 2020). "An Effective Treatment for Coronavirus (COVID-19)." Retrieved December 7, 2021, from https://docs.google.com/document/d/e/2PACX-1vTi-g18ftNZUMRAj2SwRPodtscFio7bJ7GdNgbJAGb dfF67WuRJB3ZsidgpidB2eocFHAVjIL-7deJ7/pub?fbclid=IwAROgPsui9XcTEix8PvYfKWVMX3ArYwj5AsXmxA3riSrE5_ JTxvqHyYxReHg.

91 Musk, E. (March 16, 2020). Twitter. Retrieved December 7, 2021, from https://twitter.com/elonmusk/ status/1239650597906898947?s=20.

92 Rankovic, D. (March 25, 2020). "Google censors Google Doc of medical hydroxychloroquine coronavirus treatment trial paper." Retrieved December 7, 2021, from https://reclaimthenet.org/google-censors-google-doc-hydroxychloroquine/.

obscuring the active experimental progress researchers and physicians were already making?

After a few months, Google restored Dr. Todaro's and Rigano's document, but by then the damage to the reputations of those medications and those who prescribed it was already done. At the time of this writing, early December 2020, Twitter preempts any link to that document with a manipulative "Warning: this link may be unsafe" page for anyone who clicks it. That page is written in the same style as warnings you often see on websites that contain malware. At the bottom of the warning, in small print, it says, "Ignore this warning and continue" with a link to the document on the word "continue."[93]

I've done my best to converse with others who disagree or claim to disagree with my perspective that the data on early treatment is overwhelmingly positive. I'd like to better understand all perspectives, and the people who have them. That's what it takes to solve some hard problems, and we may be facing harder problems than simply understanding evidence associated with proper medical care. In particular, I'd like to understand the well-educated professionals and academics who do not see, or claim not to see, the efficacy of early treatment regimens in the data. I believe I can identify several attributes driving their blindness.

- **Fear.** First and foremost, a campaign of terror was laid down through media, government, and the medical establishment that made people worry that they, their families, their neighborhoods,

---

93 Retrieved December 7, 2021, from https://twitter.com/safety/unsafe_link_warning?unsafe_link=https://docs.
google.com/document/d/e/2PACX-1vTi-g18ftNZUMRAj2SwRPodtscFio7bJ7GdNgbJAGbdfF67WuRJB3ZsidgpidB2eoc
FHAVjIL-7deJ7/pub.

and all of civilization might not survive the pandemonium. In a panic, people stop thinking *deliberatively*. The economics of time often dictates the effects. People still have to work and take care of their families. Not everyone can press "pause" and devote several dozen hours a week to understanding the totality of everything that happened during the pandemic. That makes it easy for accepted authority icons to dictate reality *at* them.

- **Cognitive dissonance**. The media crowns experts and can do so to project a conclusion from which to work backward to arrange the "facts." It doesn't matter if you're the world's most well-published infectious disease expert, as is Dr. Raoult. For the mass audience, that credential is meaningless if the media doesn't tell you about it. People who find themselves hypnotized by such media cannot hope to escape the illusion easily. If you are unfamiliar with the Asch conformity experiment, you may want to stop and read up on it. Even worse, many of the hypnotized are trained to attack and denigrate alternative viewpoints. That's the way narcissism works, whether natural or acquired.

- **Ambition**. Call it sociopathy if you like. People motivated by ends over means with little regard to the complex relationships between the two tend to pay great attention to and emulate those whom the media tells them are *successful*. When those people are "experts" who are in complete opposition to the use of medicine for the early treatment of COVID-19, many of the ambitious will distance themselves from anyone not found to be in complete opposition to early treatment while miming the attitudes of the anointed experts. Ambitious people do not necessarily deny scientific reasoning as a rule, but do not find most of it interesting enough to take a public position about unless it helps them in some tangible way.

- **Indoctrination**. Over the courses of their educations, some people sacrifice the practice of personal judgment to the proxy judgment of textbook methods and authorities. Such heuristic methods are generally enticing insofar as they *usually* give a better answer than throwing darts might. But religious trust in the methods leaves those indoctrinated by their educations in a highly suggestible state that can be gamed by sophisticated manipulators. Since breaking away from that state involves suffering ridicule led by the ambitious, and joined in by those who are themselves indoctrinated or suffering from cognitive dissonance, the indoctrinated are emotionally trapped without agency. They become habitually unable to exercise their own judgment without expressed permission from somewhere safe in their perceived hierarchy.
- **Projection of goodness**. People project their understanding of themselves onto the world. Good people who do not think about harming or conning other people often take longer to recognize when bad people are fooling them.

Or maybe this examination is my own masking of my misinterpretations of reality? I'm old enough at this point to always leave that question open, and some of those who disagree with me, like Professor Ioannidis, really have demonstrated excellence during their careers. Not to mention, I certainly don't disagree with all of his statements during the pandemic (such as a belief in choice in vaccination over mandates, and that lockdowns don't work). Maybe I should just trust all of his stated views?

Science is about the judgment of each observer with a thoughtfully neutral methodology, not proxy trust in experts. We can choose not to engage in science, and at times that is the economic choice. But this time the stakes are too high for that, so we must engage in scientific thinking. And for better or worse, there is no complete set of rules for how we view data or judge the results of experiments. Judgment is a skill sharpened by experience and deliberate training, and in building that skill, we come to understand reasons why some forms of evidence are generally, but maybe not always, better than others. All that we can do is to do our best.

But when I am left to my own judgment, I find *repetition* and *consistency* of scientific results to be most persuasive. Both in my work with Dr. Tyson and Dr. Fareed, and elsewhere, I have found astonishing consistency in the efficacy of early treatment—particularly from the use of hydroxychloroquine and ivermectin—to combat COVID-19.

- Dr. Tyson and Dr. Fareed: approximately 7,000 patients with four hospitalizations and zero deaths.
- Dr. Raoult: He and his colleagues have published scores of papers,[94] some of which I have read, but as best I can recall one summarized the use of hydroxychloroquine early treatment protocols applied to approximately 8,000 patients, with just five deaths, as of sometime in 2021.
- Dr. Ben Marble: Dr. Marble is the first physician to treat patients in all fifty states. He and his staff have treated 65,000 patients at the early stages of COVID-19 with what he describes as a 99.99% survival rate, meaning in the ballpark of six or seven total deaths.
- Dr. Vipul Shah: As of June 2021, Dr. Shah had lost just five out of around 8,000 patients using hydroxychloroquine during the

---

94   Mediterraneev Infection. (April 14, 2020). "PUBLICATIONS & PREPRINT IHU." Retrieved December 7, 2021, from https://www.mediterranee-infection.com/pre-prints-ihu/.

first pandemic wave in India, then ivermectin during the second. He explained to me that he switched treatment protocols due to Facebook's censoring of his communication with other physicians and patients.

- Dr. Vladimir Zelenko: Out of around 3,000 patients, only two died.
- Dr. Brian Procter: Through September 2020, Dr. Procter put 922 patients through his treatment protocol with six hospitalizations and one death.[95] I lost track of his tally after Twitter revoked his account.
- Dr. Luigi Cavanna: By April 2020, Dr. Cavanna stated in an interview with *Time* that he had treated 280 outpatients in COVID-ravaged Italy with around 5% hospitalization and zero deaths.[96] The media stopped reporting on his success, but it is noteworthy that Italy begin treating far larger numbers of outpatients, and using hydroxychloroquine for most inpatients after word of his success spread.
- Senior Clinical Pharmacist Abdulrahman Mohana: In a study of 238 outpatient fever clinics prescribing hydroxychloroquine to 2,733 COVID-19 patients in Saudi Arabia, there were no ICU admissions or deaths reported.[97]
- Dr. Heather Gessling: By September 2021, Columbia, Missouri's top-ranked family physician had treated around 1,500 patients,

95 Procter, Brian C et al. "Clinical outcomes after early ambulatory multidrug therapy for high-risk SARS-CoV-2 (COVID-19) infection." *Reviews in cardiovascular medicine* vol. 21,4 (2020): 611-614. Doi:10.31083/j.rcm.2020.04.260.

96 Berardi, F. (April 9, 2020). "The Italian Doctor Flattening the Curve by Treating COVID-19 Patients in Their Homes." *Time.* Retrieved December 7, 2021, from https://time.com/collection/coronavirus-heroes/5816874/italy-coronavirus-patients-treating-home/.

97 Mohana, Abdulrhman et al. "Hydroxychloroquine Safety Outcome within Approved Therapeutic Protocol for COVID-19 Outpatients in Saudi Arabia." *International journal of infectious diseases : IJID : official publication of the International Society for Infectious Diseases* vol. 102 (2021): 110-114. doi:10.1016/j.ijid.2020.10.031.

losing just one due to nonadherence to treatment. She was later fired as Chief of Staff from the hospital where she worked.

- Dr. John Littell: Well over 2,000 patients were treated early with around ten deaths (all Delta variant infections).
- Dr. Mollie James: Around 1,000 patients were treated, five hospitalizations (all relatively late to treatment among the early treatment patients), and zero deaths.
- Dr. Ryan Cole: Around 350 patients with zero hospitalizations and zero deaths.
- Dr. Pierre Kory: Between 150 and 200 patients with one hospitalization and zero deaths.
- Dr. Kimberly Milhoan: Around 200 were treated with a few hospitalizations and zero deaths.
- Dr. Katarina Lindley: Around 100 were treated with five hospitalizations and zero deaths.
- Dr. Deborah Chisholm: Around 100 were treated with zero deaths.

What I see in these results is *repetition*. And *consistency*. The 100,000 or so patients represented here suffered around thirty total deaths, which comes out to a 99.97% survival rate. Most of these patients were in the U.S., and the aggregate fatality rate among these patients is around 98% lower than the U.S. average, just as I had observed when aggregating global data more than a year ago. Note that the treatments prescribed among these physicians vary with some patients receiving hydroxychloroquine, some receiving ivermectin, and some receiving both medications.

Most of these doctors put on their Captain Obvious hats and give their patients vitamins and zinc, too. They prescribe corticosteroids or monoclonal antibodies where they see fit. They practice empiric medicine, using practiced judgments to fit the treatment to the patient and the symptoms present. The whole is never really the sum of the parts, so it is impossible, not to say inappropriate, to ascribe a certain proportion of this dramatic success to any one medicine, and while individual studies can sometimes confirm their success, no study of any of the treatments in isolation can logically confirm their failure in combination with the rest.

These are not the only doctors whose stories I could tell. I've communicated with several others, and heard secondhand anecdotes about many more. I do not have statistics to report for all of them. Within the numbers that I do have, the collective mortality rate is not much different from background mortality (people who would have died under normal circumstances), and while I do not know the full details, a substantial portion of the mortality is reportedly associated with nonadherence to the prescribed treatments.

Repetition. Consistency.

I have yet to talk to or even hear about a doctor who stopped providing early ambulatory treatment of COVID-19 patients after failing to keep nearly all of their patients healthy. Not one. Not from anywhere in the world after communicating with hundreds of researchers and physicians, discovering that tens or hundreds of thousands of physicians around the globe have used these early treatment medications and principles during the pandemic. Either these treatments work, or they're all physicians with previously unimpeachable careers who independently decided to lie to cover up their delusions, and without one whistleblower or shred of evidence contradicting their stories.

What else could I conclude?

Repetition. Consistency.

DID ANYONE AT ALL REALLY NEED TO DIE FROM COVID-19?

As I wrote honestly in the paper analyzing Dr. Tyson and Dr. Fareed's patient data, there are limitations to our study just as there are to all studies. First and foremost, the study is a retrospective case series. Many case series are difficult to use in making highly certain judgments. We make the best judgments we can about medicines when we can compare the outcomes from two groups of patients (cohorts) with highly similar overall risk profiles, then give medicine to one of those groups (the treatment arm) and a placebo to the other (the control arm).

It is generally difficult to fit a case series in retrospect to a proper cohort that is perfectly matched in health risks for comparison. Ordinarily, this would be done by matching individual patients with highly similar health profiles. This kind of case matching is the reason that the study of Dr. Zelenko's results included only a fraction of his patients, which I believe resulted in an underestimate of the effect size of his treatment, as well as the number of lives he saved. But case matching is not the only way to achieve cohorts with similar overall risk profiles. With respect to the goal of understanding that a medicine or medical regimen works well, we need only be certain that a cohort that represents a proper control arm *exists*, whether or not we can identify them. For this case series, the results are so profound, that Occam's razor suggests that it exists somewhere between the synthetic control groups that I compared the case series against. And if it exists in that extremely wide range of possibilities, it would imply that the protocols of Dr. Tyson and Dr. Fareed are effective in reducing disease, reducing the consumption of medical resources, and saving lives.

But in all fairness, computing an effect size like a percentage reduction in rates of hospitalization and death, are extremely difficult to do achieve perfectly from a case series—even one of exceptionally large size. Is the reduction in mortality due to early treatment as much as 97% or 98% (or maybe 99% or more once we sweep away background mortality and nonadherence rates?) as I've come to believe? If it isn't, that suggests that our case series consists of an exceptionally healthy group of individuals.

This is where the sensitivity analysis comes into play in our study. I will try to explain what that's about for readers unfamiliar with statistical analysis.

When I first analyzed the AVUC data, I looked at the age distribution profile of the AVUC patients and compared it to the Imperial County data. I adjusted for that risk before running standard computations to compare the AVUC cohort with the non-AVUC cohort. The AVUC cohort was a bit younger, with fewer patients over the age of eighty.

Without complete data for comorbidities such as diabetes rates and coronary heart disease, I made the reasonable observation that even with respect to age, nursing home patients and those confined to hospitals or hospices are at greater risk. So, the AVUC patients should be said to be at less risk than the non-AVUC patients. But by how much? This is where we run into trouble with most case series.

At some point, it struck me that the profound nature of the results allowed for me to go a step further than is typically available with a case series. If I compare the AVUC patients with the non-AVUC patients where even with a risk adjustment for age, I would likely be overestimating the effect size for hospitalizations. However, I could also imagine a subset of the 21,000 or so non-AVUC patients who did have similar health profiles to the AVUC cohort. That may sound strange because we cannot know the exact hospitalization or mortality rates of such a subset without a godlike ability to identify them. But we can ask a series of reasonable questions:

- What does the comparison look like if we reduce the risk of hospitalization and death to the results after correction for age (to 20.76% and 2.25%, respectively)?
- What does the comparison look like if we reduce the risks further to 15% and 1.5%?
- What does the comparison look like if we reduce the risks further to 10% and 1%?
- What does the comparison look like if we reduce the risks further to 5% and 0.5%?
- What are the limits of these risk reductions that still result in statistically significant results?

My personal best guess is that the perfect non-AVUC comparison group of virtually identical health profiles lies somewhere in the middle of my chosen synthetic comparison groups (fictional comparison groups with varying levels of health or immunity). That's a judgment call. I'm willing to put boundaries on it, but I will defend it with anyone who takes an honest look at the raw patient data. Maybe my guesstimate is wrong, but I'd certainly be willing to bet on it because I've seen *repetition* and *consistency* elsewhere. But what I'm *far more certain about* is that the health profiles of the AVUC patients are *far above* the answer to the last question, and that's primarily what we need to know. That means that a godlike observer could analyze the results as if through the lens of a perfectly executed RCT and conclude that AVUC's results represent a statistically significant improvement.

Why am I so certain?

1. If the perfect non-AVUC comparison group suffers 99% less hospitalization than the aggregate non-AVUC county patients, then the AVUC results still represent a statistically significant improvement.
2. If the perfect non-AVUC comparison group suffers 96% less mortality than the aggregate non-AVUC county patients, then the AVUC results still represent a statistically significant improvement.

If the COVID-19 sufferers who happened to walk through the door at AVUC were *that* much healthier than the average county residents, and in ways aside from age profile alone, then we have a truly magical mystery on our hands and we should probably declare the five AVUC clinic locations magical magnets that repel those with invisible, undiscovered attributes that make them susceptible to COVID-19.

I think I'll stick with the less extraordinary explanation, which is that the care received by AVUC patients made a difference, and we can see that clearly in the data.

The RCT fundamentalists are going to say this evidence is not convincing because it *cannot* be convincing. But their story is not about science or statistics, it's about *control*. They want to control how you think by declaring a rule that does not exist. That's part of the business model for the behemoth corporate pharmaceutical conglomerates. They want you to believe in a methodological pyramid of evidence in which RCTs are necessarily above retrospective observational studies like ours. And all other things being *equal*, they would be correct. But the idea that all other things are equal is simply wrong.

The *existence* of the near-perfect comparison group among non-AVUC COVID-19 patients in Imperial County is nearly certain, and it is far more perfect as a comparison group than could be expected from an RCT where patient sorting takes place according to algorithms using limited sets of variables. There is no god of statistical perfection running RCTs in practice, so the matching of risk factors never takes place with godlike perfection.

The gold standard of scientific experimentation is not the RCT. If there is a gold standard in science, it's *critical thinking*. Critical thinking governs the way hypotheses are formulated, experiments are designed, and results are analyzed. Critical thinking helps us understand that critical thinking is itself a variable on a different axis than methodology, which is only ever as good as its application.

At this point, you are primarily left with two possible judgments:

1. Early treatment regimens such as the ones used by all the physicians mentioned in this book substantially reduce COVID-19 disease progression and mortality.
2. That the 99.97% survival rate of the patients receiving such care tells us that the vast majority of the population has very little to worry about during this pandemic. In that case, all of the cumbersome lockdowns, masks, and experimental "vaccines" with so many red flags and unknown risks are entirely unnecessary except perhaps among high-risk patients (a still-debatable point). Stop worrying and let the kids out to play in the yard, regardless.

The wiggle room is small. Think it through.

My sincerest thanks to my heroes, Dr. Brian Tyson and Dr. George Fareed, who invited me onto these projects. These men are heroes who have stood up to ridicule in order to do the right thing in treating patients early, and with all the available tools at their disposal. Since I've gotten to know him, I've started calling Dr. Tyson "the honey badger of urgent care clinicians" for his dedication to using every available tool in the mission of saving every single patient who walks into one of his clinics. And Dr. Fareed is the epitome of the gentleman physician, which you likely understand if you've heard him speak. And if you haven't, follow the links at the end of this book to his many video testimonials delivered by his patients. If at this point that doesn't move you, nothing will.

RESOURCES

Many people are not receiving vital information about COVID treatment—which is understandable when the mainstream media has not been fully transparent about the pandemic from the start. For this reason, we want to ensure you have all the resources you need at your fingertips. This section will provide additional information related to COVID-specific telemedicine services, how to get help if you need it, and additional resources that challenge mainstream medical advice. May this information empower and enlighten you!

Dr. Fareed and Dr. Tyson are among a group of experts providing valuable help to stem the pandemic at a website for early COVID-19 care: https://earlycovidcare.org/our-expert/.

A volunteer group run by Mathew Crawford has grown to a few dozen active participants from around the world, and with a wide range of talents and professional backgrounds. They started building www.campfire.wiki to document pandemic events and research (since this cannot be expected to happen at Wikipedia).

They started a George Fareed article and dropped this video there:

https://www.campfire.wiki/doku.php?id=george_fareed

COVID-SPECIFIC TELEMEDICINE SERVICES

Many telemedicine services have been created and expanded to vastly improve the availability of early COVID-19 treatment for Americans. This has been the result of conscientious and informed doctors wanting to help those suffering all over the U.S. and beyond in this pandemic. These websites focused on treatment and prevention using hydroxychloroquine, ivermectin, nutraceuticals, while using many different protocols, including Dr. Zelenko's, FLCC, the AFLDS, as well as our own plans for treatment and prophylaxis.

We resolved we were not going to allow our patients to go home alone, without treatment or understanding what this virus was and what to expect. Instead, we (along with other physicians from around the nation) grouped together and created telemedicine sites so people could call and receive the answers they deserved.

The sites below have seen tens of thousands of patients each month, because too many conventional offices and urgent cares across the country continued to operate as if there were no available outpatient treatments:

https://myfreedoctor.com/
https://speakwithanmd.com/
https://americasfrontlinedoctors.org/
https://synergyhealthdpc.com/covid-care/
www.covidoutpatientcare.com
www.silverstrandurgentcare.com

FREE E-BOOK

This e-book, based on Dr. Zelenko's method, details the principles of early antiviral treatment. To read this invaluable resource, *Medical Studies Support MD's Prescribing Hydroxychloroquine for Early Stage COVID-19 and for Prophylaxis*, click here: https://files.internetprotocol. co/ebook-covid19.pdf

BOOKS:

The Real Anthony Fauci: Bill Gates, Big Pharma, and the Global War on Democracy and Public Health (Children's Health Defense)
Robert F. Kennedy Jr.

COVID-19 and the Global Predators: We Are the Prey
Peter R. Breggen, M.D. and Ginger Ross Breggen

Ivermectin for Freedom
Justus R. Hope

Ivermectin for the World
Justus R. Hope

VALUABLE VIDEOS:

Building on the theme of his recent best-selling book, *The Real Anthony Fauci*, Robert Kennedy, Jr. delivered his clear and honest pleas for people (citizens) throughout the world to reclaim their rights and overcome the oppression (totalitarian) of the last twenty-one months for the sake of humanity and the pandemic injustices. (November 13, 2021, in Italy.)

https://www.bitchute.com/video/WcB9Bm61MYE6/

Dr. Peter McCullough, a prominent cardiologist and COVID-19 authority who has been published in hundreds of acclaimed medical journals, discuses the suppression of information regarding serious adverse reactions to the genetic COVID-19 vaccines and about vaccine mandates.

https://steadfastclash.com/the-latest/watch-top-cardiologist-discusses-shocking-study-regarding-jab-vs-virus/

In this video from COVEXIT, Dr. Risch discusses the rationale for outpatient early treatment, the scientific evidence that early treatment is safe and effective, the pros and cons of randomized controlled trials, how to prevent outbreaks in nursing homes, and the role of prophylaxis:

https://youtu.be/cf3_YXR70Ug

Dr. Tyson spoke at a Freedom Rally on November 8, 2021, about natural immunity, your rights regarding vaccines that are not FDA-approved (but instead are operating under an EUA), the case for not vaccinating healthy children, and the benefits of early COVID treatment. You can access the video here:

https://m.facebook.com/ImperialValleyCitizensAgainstMandates/videos/339127887971379/?refsrc=deprecated&_rdr

Below is a link to an article and video that covers a recent public speech given by Tyson and Fareed on December 21, 2021, that triggered

COVID-19 misinformation by agencies and individuals. Despite several requests to remove the item from the meeting, the Imperial County Board of Supervisors heard from Dr. George Fareed and Dr. Brian Tyson at the regular meeting Tuesday, December 21, regarding their COVID-19 treatment protocol. See their full presentation and more:

https://roundingtheearth.substack.com/p/the-art-of-gaslighting-argument-by

Featured in this video is an in-depth interview with the Robert Malone, M.D., the physician who discovered mRNA technology, detailing pandemic truths which must be recognized and are important components of our work in this book.

https://open.spotify.com/episode/3SCsueX2bZdbEzRtKOCEyT?si=OedIgv5VQqiPqZ2RfrrvCg

This video, with English subtitles, is of a recent seminar showing brilliant work of how variants evolve in vaccinated populations to preserve ADE epitopes (antibody dependent enhancement = facilitators for infection) and lose the NDE epitopes (neutralization epitopes):

https://www.youtube.com/watch?app=desktop&v=wBm1BKL4zlg.

TESTIMONIALS

Throughout this book, we have provided a glimpse into the lives of those touched by—and recovered from—COVID-19. Below you will find additional testimonials to support the incredible success of the early C19 treatment protocol so that you can rest assured that odds are in your favor of returning to a life of normalcy, even after a positive COVID diagnosis.

https://twitter.com/GeorgeFareed2/status/1416097244911071235?s=20

https://twitter.com/GeorgeFareed2/status/1412888603277991936?s=20

https://twitter.com/GeorgeFareed2/status/1411014988458721281?s=20

https://twitter.com/GeorgeFareed2/status/1400229075277389828?s=20

https://twitter.com/GeorgeFareed2/status/1399968967897141248?s=20

https://twitter.com/GeorgeFareed2/status/1388214232336900098?s=20

https://twitter.com/GeorgeFareed2/status/1387514467039145986?s=20

https://twitter.com/GeorgeFareed2/status/1386759293127467010?s=20

https://twitter.com/GeorgeFareed2/status/1386738274283126786?s=20

https://twitter.com/GeorgeFareed2/status/1384937560829476866?s=20

https://twitter.com/GeorgeFareed2/status/1381126875997560833?s=20

https://twitter.com/GeorgeFareed2/status/1379255162871586816?s=20

https://twitter.com/GeorgeFareed2/status/1379160638757367808?s=20

https://twitter.com/GeorgeFareed2/status/1377026441188044801?s=20

https://twitter.com/GeorgeFareed2/status/1376953613616959491?s=20

https://twitter.com/GeorgeFareed2/status/1374885941907660805?s=20

https://twitter.com/GeorgeFareed2/status/1374460533584228359?s=20

https://twitter.com/GeorgeFareed2/status/1374109830110060545?s=20

https://twitter.com/GeorgeFareed2/status/1374110516797272065?s=20

https://twitter.com/GeorgeFareed2/status/1373016846463463425?s=20

https://twitter.com/GeorgeFareed2/status/1373015755218776065?s=20

https://twitter.com/GeorgeFareed2/status/1372983574375239680?s=20

https://twitter.com/GeorgeFareed2/status/1372959036073598982?s=20

https://twitter.com/GeorgeFareed2/status/1372960900575940608?s=20

https://twitter.com/GeorgeFareed2/status/1372390642685333505?s=20

https://twitter.com/GeorgeFareed2/status/1372389458239123456?s=20

https://twitter.com/GeorgeFareed2/status/1372385144187752453?s=20

https://twitter.com/GeorgeFareed2/status/1372386272497438727?s=20

https://twitter.com/GeorgeFareed2/status/1372249652288835585?s=20

https://twitter.com/GeorgeFareed2/status/1372250365521915904?s=20

https://twitter.com/GeorgeFareed2/status/1372223870447484930?s=20

https://twitter.com/GeorgeFareed2/status/1372224849922326532?s=20

https://twitter.com/GeorgeFareed2/status/1369732979602329600?s=20

https://twitter.com/GeorgeFareed2/status/1369430942570471440?s=20

https://twitter.com/GeorgeFareed2/status/1369432601472155659?s=20

https://twitter.com/GeorgeFareed2/status/1369422457602514945?s=20

https://twitter.com/GeorgeFareed2/status/1369428643945021451?s=20

https://twitter.com/GeorgeFareed2/status/1367898440487735298?s=20

https://twitter.com/GeorgeFareed2/status/1367243882228981760?s=20

https://twitter.com/GeorgeFareed2/status/1364685037963120644?s=20

https://twitter.com/GeorgeFareed2/status/1364682023579779073?s=20

https://twitter.com/GeorgeFareed2/status/1361867813032366082?s=20

https://twitter.com/GeorgeFareed2/status/1361845099248848896?s=20

https://twitter.com/GeorgeFareed2/status/1361442547185291265?s=20

https://twitter.com/GeorgeFareed2/status/1361380444416081926?s=20

https://twitter.com/GeorgeFareed2/status/1359223645323730944?s=20

https://twitter.com/GeorgeFareed2/status/1357760005710127104?s=20

TESTIMONIALS

https://twitter.com/GeorgeFareed2/status/1357028952854851590?s=20

https://twitter.com/GeorgeFareed2/status/1357018519729102848?s=20

https://twitter.com/GeorgeFareed2/status/1356318372921659393?s=20

https://twitter.com/GeorgeFareed2/status/1356314694613561345?s=20

https://twitter.com/GeorgeFareed2/status/1354584684714319874?s=20

https://twitter.com/GeorgeFareed2/status/1354544957390942208?s=20

https://twitter.com/GeorgeFareed2/status/1353757508418957312?s=20

https://twitter.com/GeorgeFareed2/status/1352071327302123521?s=20

https://twitter.com/GeorgeFareed2/status/1352072352956203008?s=20

https://twitter.com/GeorgeFareed2/status/1352029864618983425?s=20

https://twitter.com/GeorgeFareed2/status/1350230918837899265?s=20

https://twitter.com/GeorgeFareed2/status/1350159128119808000?s=20

https://twitter.com/GeorgeFareed2/status/1349407956031270914?s=20

https://twitter.com/GeorgeFareed2/status/1349122463427297281?s=20

https://twitter.com/GeorgeFareed2/status/1341987498868711424?s=20

https://twitter.com/GeorgeFareed2/status/1333969469371138049?s=20

https://twitter.com/GeorgeFareed2/status/1333606552146612224?s=20

https://twitter.com/georgefareed2/status/1421194585854803968?s=21

https://twitter.com/GeorgeFareed2/status/1461767893847187456?s=20